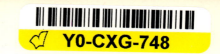

ZEN YOGA THERAPY

Zen Yoga Therapy

by Masahiro Oki

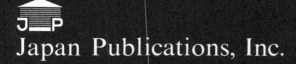
Japan Publications, Inc.

Published by JAPAN PUBLICATIONS, INC., Tokyo

Distributors:
UNITED STATES: *Kodansha International/USA, Ltd., through Harper & Row, Publishers, Inc., 10 East 53rd Street, New York, New York 10022.* SOUTH AMERICA: *Harper & Row, Publishers, Inc., International Department.* CANADA: *Fitzhenry & Whiteside Ltd., 150 Lesmill Road, Don Mills, Ontario M3B 2T6.* MEXICO AND CENTRAL AMERICA: *HARLA S. A. de C. V., Apartado 30–546, Mexico 4, D. F.* BRITISH ISLES: *International Book Distributors Ltd., 66 Wood Lane End, Hemel Hempstead, Herts HPZ 4RG.* EUROPEAN CONTINENT: *Boxerbooks, Inc., Limmatstrasse 111, 8031 Zurich.* AUSTRALIA AND NEW ZEALAND: *Book Wise (Australia) Pty. Ltd., 104–8 Sussex Street, Sydney 2000.* THE FAR EAST AND JAPAN: *Japan Publications Trading Co., Ltd., 1–2–1, Sarugaku-cho, Chiyoda-ku, Tokyo 101.*

First edition: October 1979

LCCC No. 79–1960
ISBN 0–87040–459–8

Printed in Japan

Introduction

Yoga does not interpret health and illness as opposites. Instead, it considers illness to be a manifestation of life's movement in the direction of regeneration of health; that is, a natural solution to abnormalities. Consequently, in the Yoga view, co-operation with the natural operations of life can cure sickness. Unnatural things that impair the operations of life force, on the other hand, cause illness. In my own long history of combating illness and of research in therapy, I have learned that cures must be both physical and mental and must arise from within the living organism: they cannot be effected by means of total reliance on outside agencies. The evil conditions that bring about sickness are as follows:
1. Abnormal posture and movements,
2. Abnormal and insufficient nourishment,
3. Emotional imbalance and insecurity,
4. Confusion, excessive attachments to things and people, and misunderstandings,
5. Abnormalities and strains at work, at home, or in the general environment.

Obstructions to the normal functioning of life force manifest themselves in the forms of individual symptoms, which are expressions of the self-curative, self-regulating operations of life. If they are not smoothly eliminated and corrected, chronic illness develops.

The Yoga therapeutic system cooperates with the operation of life force by means of deliberate efforts to correct irregularities in posture, motion, dietary habits, and psychological conditions. No matter what the sickness, correction of the conditions causing it stimulates natural powers of recuperation. True health is a state in which powers to correct and eliminate pathological conditions operate regularly and without hitch.

Yoga includes ways of actively correcting illness, ways of curing by allowing natural recuperation to take place, and ways to allow cures to be effected without deliberate steps. Similarly, in relation to good health, Yoga has deliberate methods for promoting it, deliberate ways of allowing it to develop on its own, and ways of allowing it to emerge without deliberate acts. I term the method in which steps are taken to effect a cure therapeutic; the way in which cures are allowed to develop on their own, natural; and the method of allowing the cure to develop without seeking it, religious. In the establishment of good health, the first system is a set of techniques, the second a set of rules, and the third a set of philosophical-religious regimens.

The passive Yoga psychosomatic therapeutic system is a natural method; the active one is a religious method. Yoga applies therapeutic techniques according to the case in hand and, from the standpoint of therapy as well as health, can be said to include all of Eastern and Western medicine and in some respects to surpass both.

My method is not an instant way to good health, but a method for psychosomatic purification (or natural recovery). All three kinds of excercises—corrective, fundamental, and strengthening—must be performed if true good health is to be maintained. In time of sickness, if exercises other than the ones considered necessary to the cure are added to the regimen, recovery will be faster; and there will be no after symptoms. Although actually the total corrective system must include consideration of posture, motion, diet, and mental state, it is impossible to cover all these elements in the limits of this one book.

Yoga is physical training for the sake of mental development. Here I shall say only that physical recovery is a temporary change unless the mental state is improved.

In this book, I include my special systems for beauty cure and for natural childbirth. The many beauty regimens popular in many parts of the world today are unnatural. If they sometimes produce temporary improvements, they are always accompanied by after symptoms. A person who is healthy is beautiful. A person who is not beautiful is either unhealthy or suffering from some unnatural condition. Zen Yoga attempts to correct individual abnormalities and to restore and maintain true beauty. Since my system eliminates all things that impair the natural normal operations of life force, a person who performs these exercises regularly finds that medicines are more effective and that, should it become necessary, surgery is successful.

In conclusion, I should like to emphasize an important point. Yoga is a total psychosomatic system. This book deals with such physical aspects as breathing exercises and calisthenics only. Consequently, the reader must not rely on it entirely.

Contents

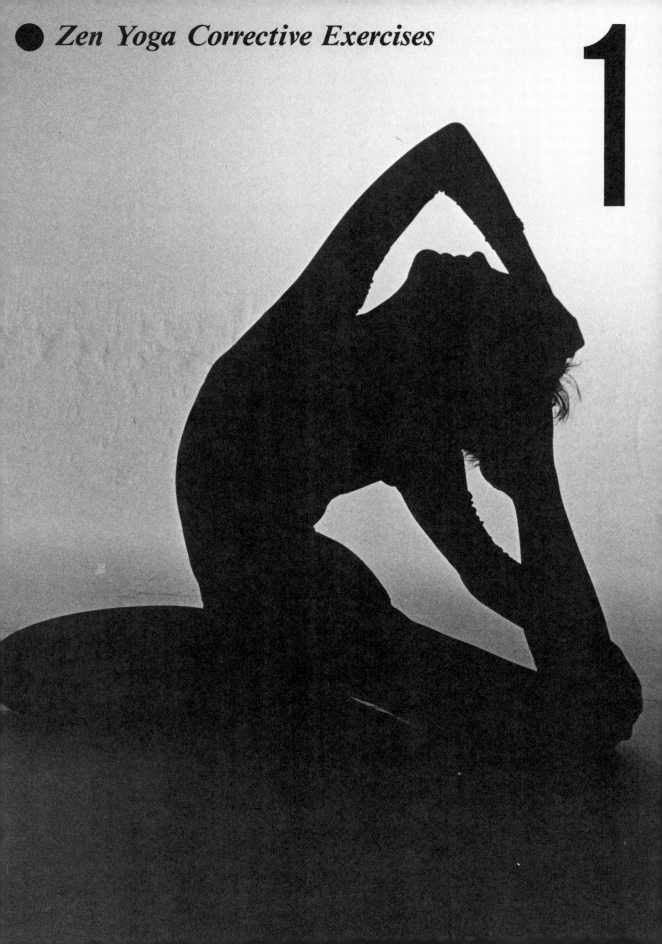

● *Zen Yoga Corrective Exercises*

1

About Yoga

Yoga attempts to select the truly useful from the many things that are said to be beneficial to life. In the Yoga training hall, various health regimens are examined, and their effects are judged in the attempt to find out what is true and what is false and to produce a general synthesis of the true. The good parts of various regimens are extracted and included in Yoga exercises designed to produce over-all improvements. Some health plans actually lower body strength because, concentrating only on one part of the physical system and stimulating only parts of the body, they cause abnormalities. The Yoga system, however, if performed in the right way, including both poses and meditation, is a complete system of the entire human organism.

Adopting the basic attitude that human beings are innately healthy, Yoga interprets illness as the body's way of correcting what is wrong and of restoring sound health. Since life force works by balanced adaptations and adjustments, abnormality in one system invariably causes an opposition reaction in another system. This balanced operation of life is in itself a corrective method for the restoration of good physical condition. Consequently, Yoga never treats ill people with kid gloves. On the contrary, persons who are sick must act more healthy than the healthy and must approach Yoga as if it were a matter of religious service if they expect to be cured of their ailments through it. The Yoga health plan is to bring joy to life by devising ways to enable ill people to live in a way more healthy than that of the healthy.

Yoga teaches that life is good and that, since we are all mutually valuable entities, we should live a long time. It further insists that each person is born an individual with an individual, specific mission. A person who understand this knows why he was born and how he should live.

The Yoga secret for maximum health is living in a way that brings joy to the very force of life itself, thus enabling the individual human being to manifest his own abilities to the full and to cooperate with others. A way of life in which the self and the other find satisfaction is the basic rule for health, therapy, and long life.

Yoga Corrective Exercises

Curing a physical abnormality demands understanding of over-all harmony in the organism. Though physical entities like other animals, human beings have psychological and spiritual aspects. Yoga tends to emphasize man's psychological (Buddha) nature and his daily-life elements. Occidental medicine deals very effectively with symptoms by examining the pathological condition and prescribing medicines or other treatment, including surgery, to combat it. Viewing life as a fluid phenomenon, oriental medicine alters therapeutic methods in accordance with alterations of the pathological condition. Yoga includes the good points of occidental and oriental medicine while going beyond both to produce a total system that takes into consideration individual psychological conditions and life styles.

Yoga corrective exercises are more basic, more generalized, more stage-organized, and more comprehensive than anything in the medical sciences of East or West. All of them are designed to avoid relying on outside agencies. Their major goal is to develop a body that can cooperate in the higher development of the Buddha nature inherent in all human beings. Doing this inevitably entails putting the body's physiological functions—especially those of the autonomic nervous systems—in good order. The method of achieving this aim is to strengthen the abdomen—without reliance on outside agencies.

Meaning and goal
The goal of Yoga is not merely the correction of psychosomatic abnormalities, but

also elimination of distortions and aberrations and imbalance from the whole system and stimulation of smooth operations of natural, innate, balance-maintaining powers. Conditions causing aberrations and imbalance result in personal habits and psychological inclinations that interfere with natural stability and the manifestation of the powers of life force.

Yoga Corrective Breathing Exercises

Meaning and Goal
The goal of Yoga corrective breathing exercises—one of the series including general calisthenics, dietary rules, mental exercises, and life-style regulations—improve the general psychosomatic condition. In ill persons—especially chronically ill persons—postures, motions, and breath control of the kind required for normal (natural) health are dulled. The Yoga corrective exercises consciously develop postures, motions, and breathing that are unconsciously maintained in normal, healthy people.

Effects
As long as balance is maintained in the cycle of mental tension and relaxation, the body operates normally. But, when aberrations or unequal stimulations occur, the nervous system fails to function properly, the brain works abnormally, and mental balance becomes difficult to preserve. When this happens, the body must expend excessive energy to remain balanced; and, even if illness does not develop, the person tires easily and weakens. The distortions occurring in the body cannot stimulate the suitable braking action, and the body is therefore led toward sickness. Yoga corrective breathing exercises remove aberrations and inequalities, improve natural blood circulation and the operation of the endocrine and nervous systems, give the muscles flexibility and tone, and

regulate the skeletal system. These effects, in turn, deepen the breathing and improve natural powers of recovery and the ability to relax. A person who performs Yoga corrective breathing exercises beforehand will find that he does better in work, sports, or study.

The Yoga Beauty Cure

The Zen Yoga beauty cure is an application of the corrective exercises and is totally unlike the many Yoga systems and diets currently popular all over the world. These systems are not only completely erroneous, but also, in many cases, potentially fatal if conducted even slightly incorrectly. I have evolved this beauty cure to rectify this situation.

According to the Zen Yoga system, in order for a person to be beautiful, the entire personality including its psychological, physical, and life-style aspects, must be beautiful. In other words, total balance brings true loveliness. The natural is beautiful, and ugliness is the outcome of mental and physical abnormality. Many of the so-called beauty systems do no more than alter a shape or make superficial changes without curing the abnormality. But the Zen Yoga beauty cure removes the cause of the abnormality and thus promotes true, lasting loveliness. The method is called a beauty *cure* because it eliminates the abnormality and allows the person to be beautiful in a natural way.

Performing the Exercises (1)

Though the corrective Yoga poses may look like other calisthenics, they are quite different, since their major aim is to change the breathing and in this way bring about internal alterations in the body. They are a self-control system for influencing the subconscious level of awareness by changing the conscious level. Coughing, sneezing, and yawning are natural method unconsciously applied by the body to correct something faulty. Yoga corrective exercises are consciously performed to evoke internal pressures. They must be performed accurately in a meditative state. The mind must be calm as in active Zen, and the breathing must be regulated to cause internal change and in this way to restore the body to its most natural and relaxed state.

Exercises must be used in accordance with the nature of the desired change. Once the change has been effected, other exercises must be used, for continuing to perform the same exercises not only reduced the effectiveness of the therapy, but also can do harm.

The exercises work from the outside inward. To increase their effectiveness, combine them with corrective dietary and mental regimens, which work from the inside outward. The two kinds of therapy will mutually reinforce and amplify each other. Performing the exercises before mealtime will help you to eat only what your body needs. Dietary control will assist in breathing correctly and in executing the exercises easily. The exercises will increase the effectiveness of such therapeutic methods as acupuncture and *shiatsu*. Furthermore, following each session with self-control meditation will help make the Yoga corrective regimen more meaningful and useful.

The exercises in this book are basic ones requiring the addition of specialized ones to suit the needs of the individual. They should be varied to suit the condition and the time in order to help restore the body to natural condition.

Performing the Exercises (2)

Preparations
The exercises should be performed from two to four hours after mealtime, when the stomach is empty. Go to the toilet before beginning. Clothing should be comfortable, and you should remove wristwatches, jewelry, and eyeglasses. Perform some light warming-up exercises and assume the relaxation pose for a few minutes. Deliberately yawn and stretch.

Breathing
Throughout the exercises, breathing must be deep. Inhale deeply and exhale forcefully. Breathing must be rhythmically coordinated with movement. (For instance, when you are raising and lowering your feet, inhale on the lift and exhale on the lowering motion.) Long exhalation improves powers of concentration and the ability to relax. Furthermore, it adjusts the ribs and increases their elasticity.

Mental attitude
Enjoy the exercises and be mentally relaxed about them. Do not try to get them finished in a hurry and do not be concerned solely about their effects. Smile and take advantage of the good feeling they generate.

Movements
Execute all movements accurately in accordance with the directions and with your strength deliberately concentrated in your abdomen. Always be aware of the specific point of stimulation for each exercise. If you do not, they will fail to have effect.

Perform them all to the limit of your ability. Stretch as far as you can; when instructed to tense a part of the body, put as much force in the tensing as is possible. Complete tension followed by complete relaxation will increase your powers of balance. Perform difficult movements carefully, and cautiously. Not the motion itself, but the way the effort you expend stimulates breathing, muscles, and skeleton is important. Extend the Achilles' tendons in all motions performed lying on your back.

Relaxation

At the completion of each exercise, always assume the relaxation pose for two or three minutes and put your breathing in order. Since reactions occur during the relaxation phase, failure to perform it correctly greatly reduces the effectiveness of the exercise. The body's power to correct aberrations works best when the mind and the body are relaxed. At the conclusion of the session, assume the relaxation pose for a long time.

Number of repetitions

Consult your own physical condition at the beginning of each session to determine the number of times to repeat the exercises. As a rule of thumb, from two to seven times is an average; but perform those that are difficult more times—since you need more work on them—and those that are easy fewer times. Be more deliberate and completely aware in performing the difficult exercises.

Conduct three sessions daily—morning, evening, and night—repeating the difficult exercises over and over until they become easy. When you reach this stage, reduce the number of repetitions.

Reaction phenomenon

Performing the Zen Yoga corrective exercises produces a number of reactions. You will sleep better and feel generally lighter. Some people, however, experience pain in parts of the body, feel sleepy, belch, cough, suffer from accumulation of phlegm, and undergo other apparently abnormal changes. These are all passing phenomena caused by activation of formerly paralyzed nerves and the body's attempts to correct real abnormalities. These phenomena can vary in a day's time; and, if you persevere, they will go away.

● *Preparatory Exercises*

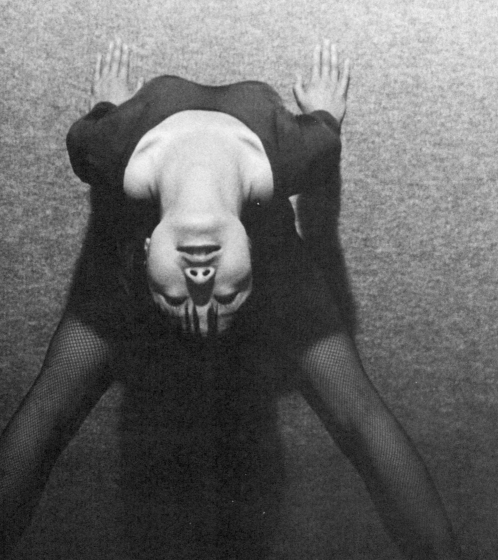

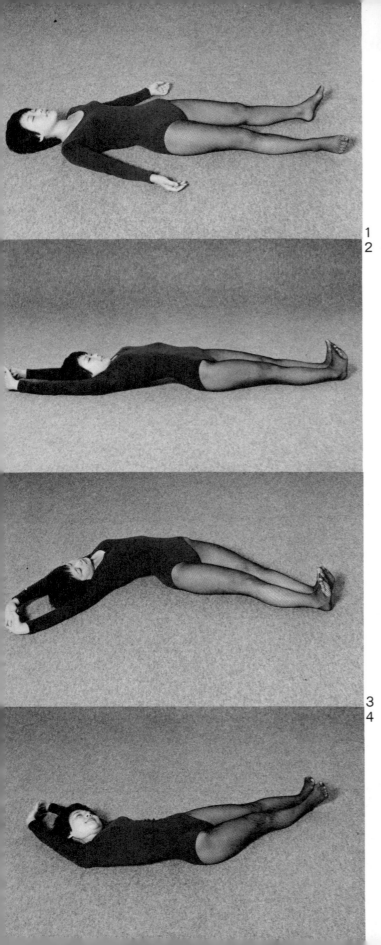

Relaxation Pose

◀ **Movements and breathing order**

1. Lying on your back, spread your arms and legs to angles of about thirty degrees to the body and incline your chin to an angle of about fifteen degrees. Letting your mouth fall open naturally, relax your entire body. Have the feeling that you have cast your weight on the floor. The palms of your hand should be turned upward.

Deliberately breathe in a deep, rhythmical fashion. Each exhalation should suggest even further relaxation.

2–4. Lock your hands together, palms turned outward, over your head and stretch your body upward and downward. Yawn and extend your Achilles' tendons while doing this. Bend your body right and left as if you were extending your rib cage. Exhale while doing this.

Execute this exercise before and after all others.

Movements and breathing order ▶

1. Lying on your back, as you exhale, raise and extend your right arm; then lower and extend your left arm. Inhaling then exhaling, extend your right arm and left leg. Your Achilles' tendons remain extended throughout this exercise.

2. Repeat with the opposite arm and leg.

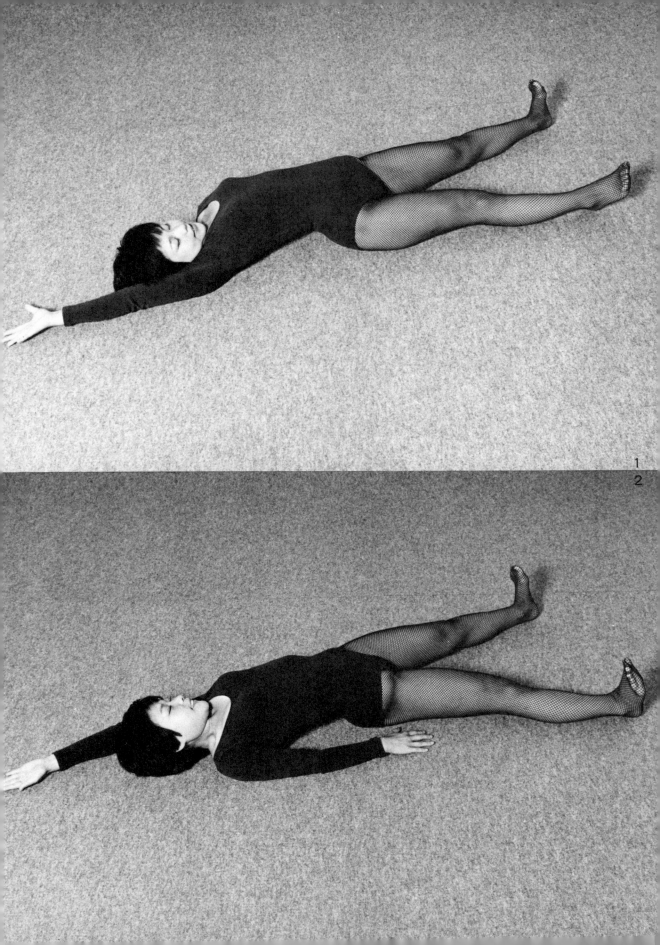

1
2

1.   Lying on your backs and keeping your elbows on the floor, bring your fore-arms—with fists clenched—upward to chest level.

2.   Extending your Achilles' tendons, inhale as you tense and raise your hips off the floor. Suddenly exhale and allow your hips to relax and drop to the floor. Repeat this exercise several times.

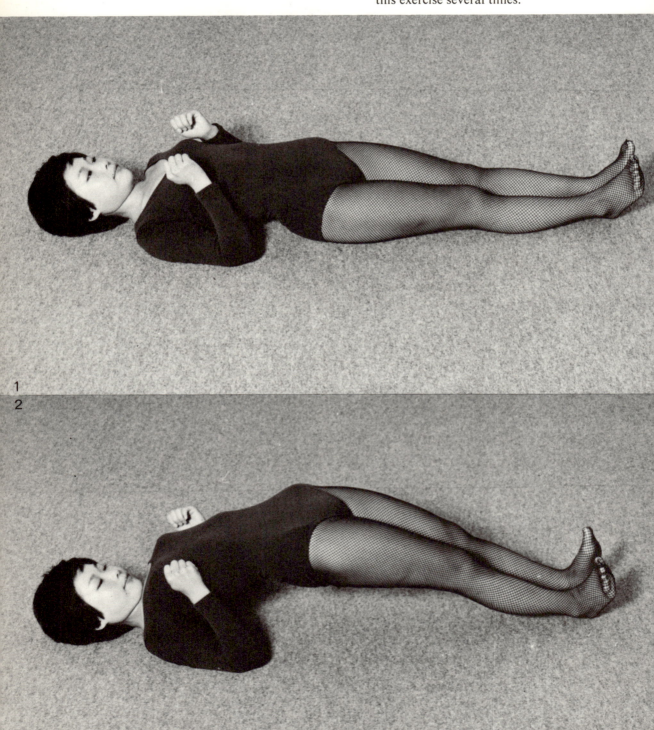

1

2

Movements and breathing order

1.   Lying on your back, raise both hands to your armpits.

2.   As you exhale, slide both elbows upward and raise your trunk so that your abdomen thrusts forward. This involves tensing the entire body. Extend your Achilles' tendons. When they are fully extended suddenly relax your whole body. Repeat this exercise several times.

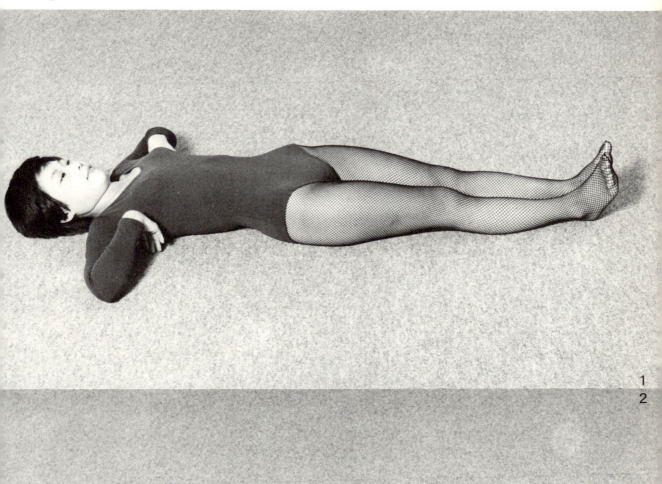

1

2

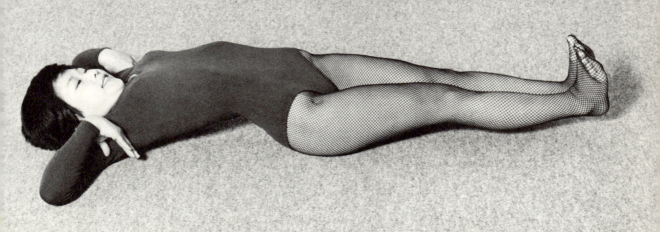

Movements and breathing order

1. Lying on your back, lock the fingers of both hands together behind your neck.

2–3. Inhale and, as you exhale, tuck your chin inward and raise and pull your head to the right, as if it were a cork you are pulling from a bottle. Your Achilles' tendons should be extended throughout this movement. Repeat in the opposite direction.

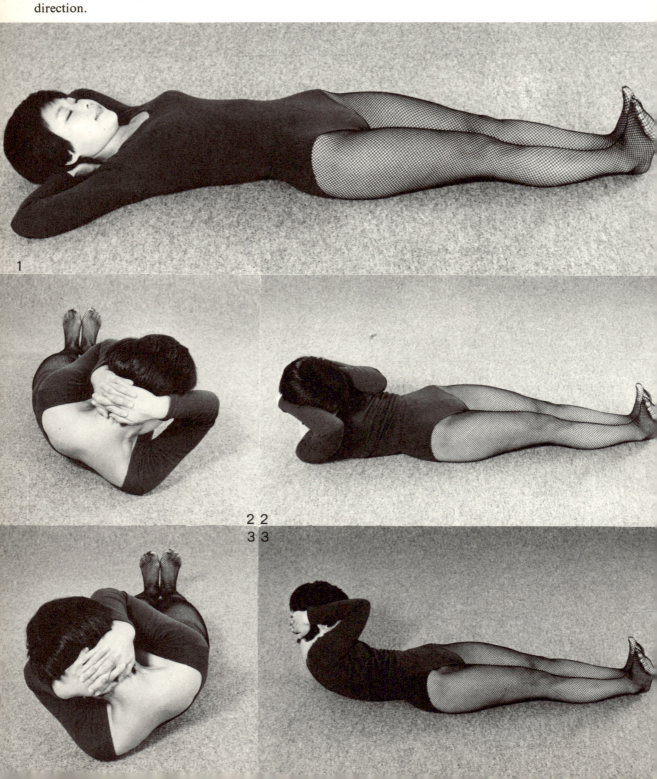

Movements and breathing order

1–4.   Yawn and stretch your body in any direction or way that feels good, as you do in the morning when you have just wakened. This is done to enable you to execute the completed relaxation pose on p. 16.

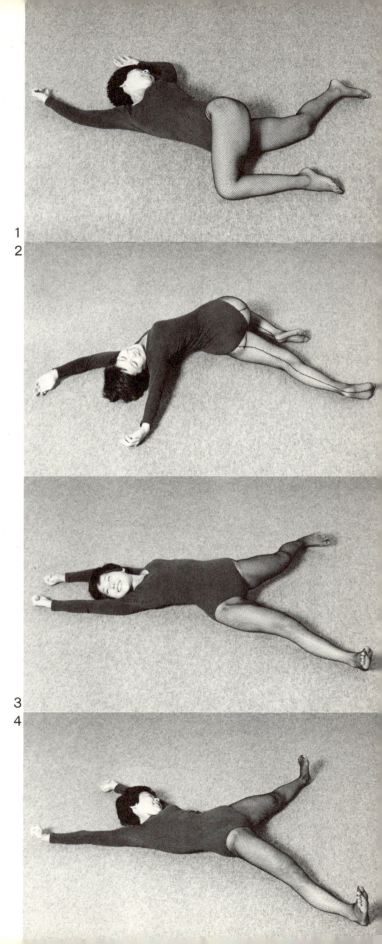

1

2

3

4

Laughing Method

Laughing is one of the best ways to counter the stresses and unpleasantnesses accompanying the daily lives of many people in modern society. It promotes ideal breathing by causing relaxation of the shoulders and neck and tensing of the abdomen and hip region. Since it is a psychosomatic control method, laughing is highly therapeutic. By bringing about a rich intake of oxygen and building up stomach pressure, it improves circulation of the blood to all parts of the body. This in turn has the invigorating effect of stimulating the functioning of the nervous and endocrine systems. You will find that performing all kinds of motions, as shown in the photographs, while deliberately laughing out loud has a refreshing and pleasant physical and mental effect.

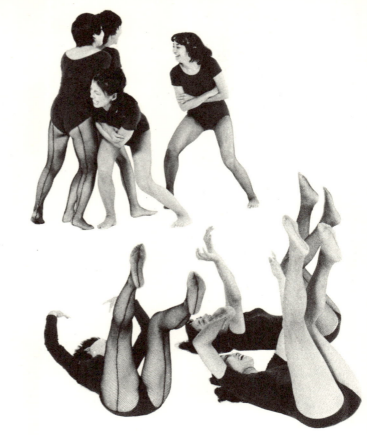

Lying supine and kicking the legs and waving the arms.

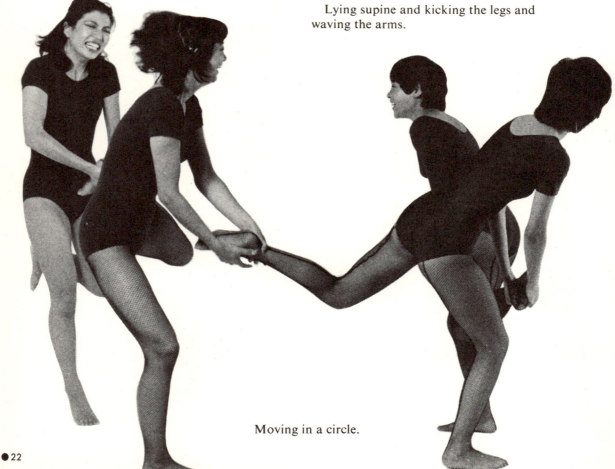

Moving in a circle.

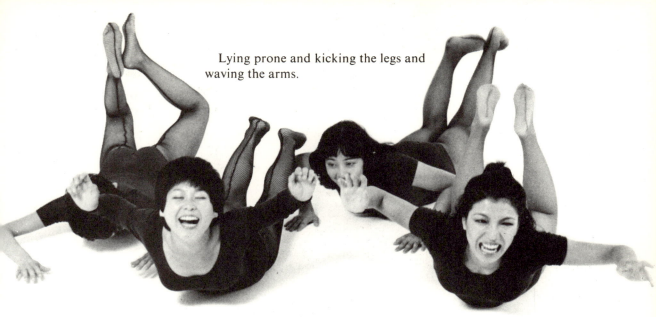

Lying prone and kicking the legs and waving the arms.

Bumping into each other with arms crossed in front of the chest.

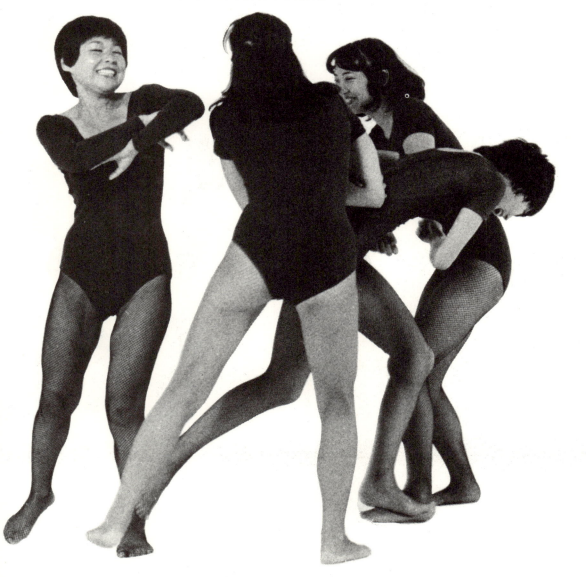

Unification

Worshipful Movements with Hands in the Prayer Attitude

Purpose and effects

The movements of this exercise are based on the position some people assume when worshipping the sun or when offering prayers in front of a temple. To execute it, the mind must be at ease and calm as if in respectful search for union with a deity. The breath must be ordered, and the entire body in harmony.

The effects of the exercise are general. It corrects right-left balance, extends muscles that tend to overcontract (for instance those of the underside of the foot), and adjusts the spine and ribs on both sides by repeated forward and rearward bends. In this way, it stabilizes the autonomous nervous system. Repeated executions of this exercise calm the mind and contribute to spiritual concentration.

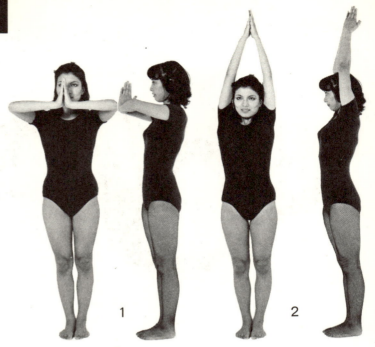

Movements and breathing order

1. With the toes of both feet aligned, stand straight and bring your hands together in the prayer attitude directly in front of your face. Pulling your chin in and extending the muscles of neck and back, tense the inner sides of your knees and your thumbs as you adjust your breathing.

Your forearms must be perfectly horizontal and your elbows at shoulder height. Tense your middle fingers and press them together. The tips of your middle fingers should be at eye level.

2–3. As you inhale, raise your joined hands high over your head and lean rearward. Your elbows must be fully extended.

4–6. Exhaling, raise your trunk to the standing position. Then slowly, with extended arms coming no farther forward than the back of your head, slowly bend forward until your palms are flat on the floor beside your feet and your head lightly touches your shins. Do not bend your knees.

7–8. Leaving your right foot in its present position and inhaling, extend your left foot well to the rear. Only the toes of your left foot should touch the floor. The knee must remain off the floor. Your weight is on your right foot, and your

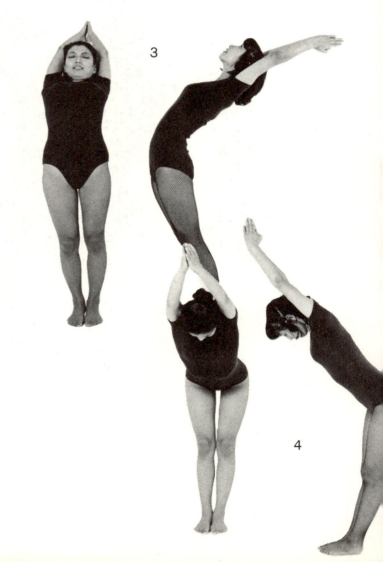

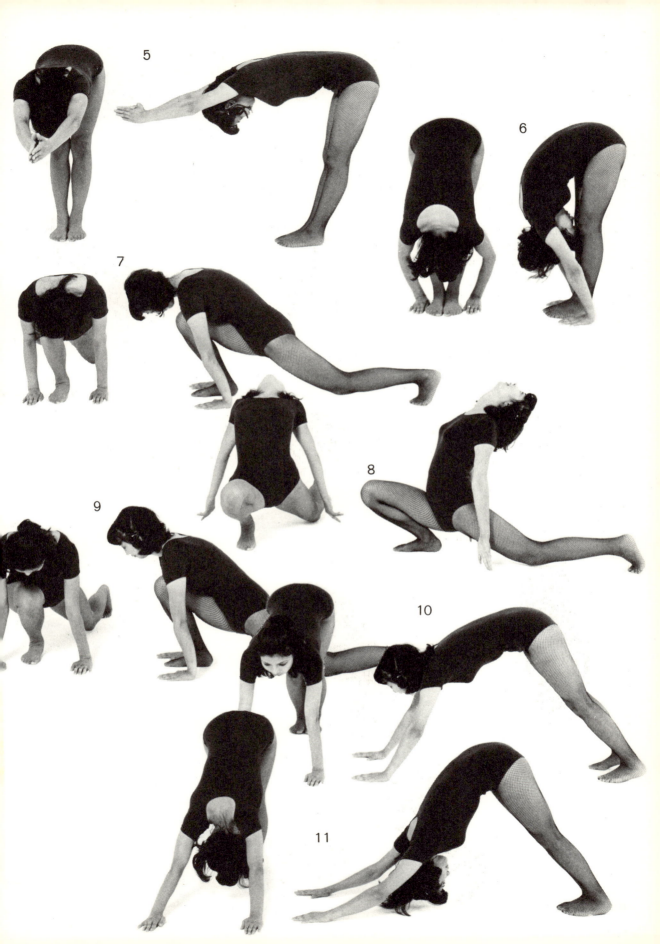

right heel remains on the floor. Raise your trunk, throw your head back, open your arms, and thrust your chest well forward.

With palms outward, your arms should open to thirty degrees to either side of your body.

9–11. Exhale as you return your hands to the floor to the sides of your right foot. Draw your right foot rearward to your left foot and raise your hips high. With knees fully extended, bring your head downward between your arms to put your body in a triangular, peaklike form. Your heels must remain on the floor.

12–13. As you inhale, bring your trunk and head forward. Leaving your right foot in the rearward position, bring your left foot forward and shift your weight to it. Then, raise your body as you did in steps 7–8.

14–15. Repeating the motions of steps 9–11, as you exhale, assume the peaklike form and return your left foot rearward to its position next to the right one.

16–17. As you inhale, lower your chest to the floor. Then, lowering your hip region to the floor too, move your body forward. Next raise and bend your trunk and head to the rear.

18. Exhaling, lower your trunk until your forehead rests on the floor. Adjust your breathing.

19. Sliding your hands about ten centimeters forward, slightly raise your hips.

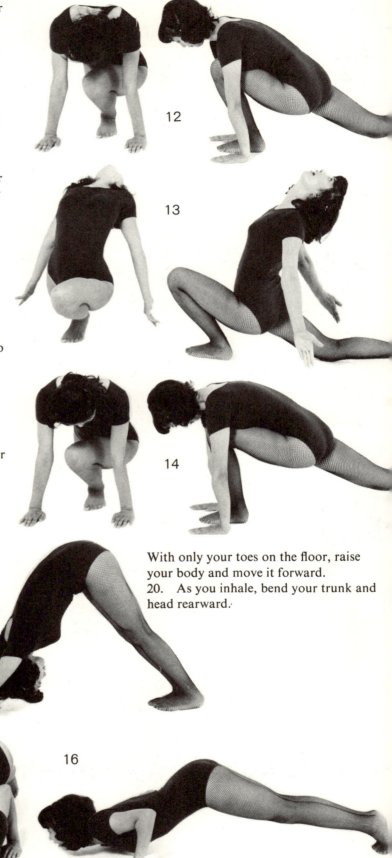

12

13

14

With only your toes on the floor, raise your body and move it forward.

20. As you inhale, bend your trunk and head rearward.

15

16

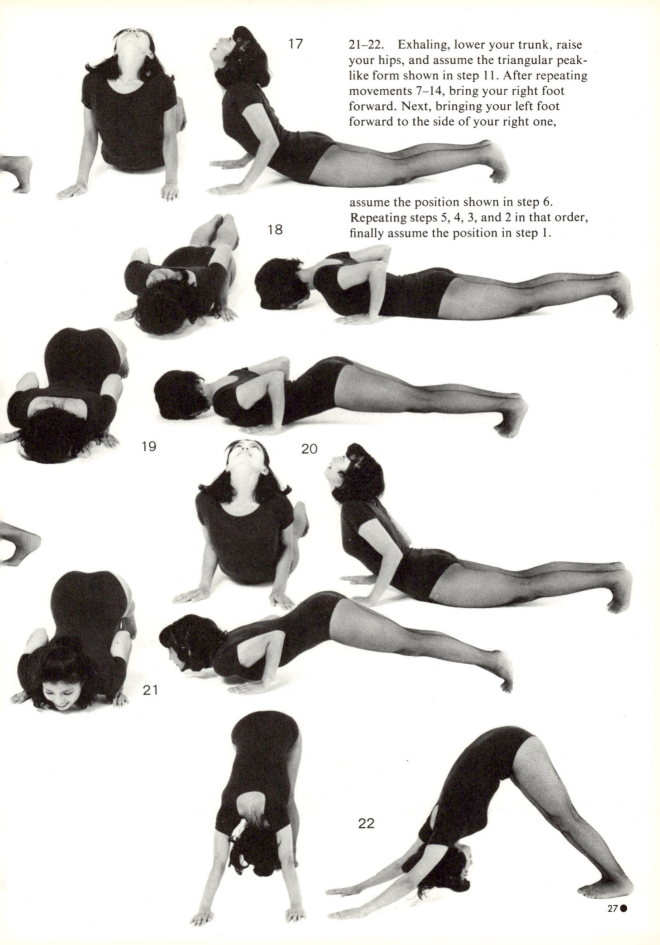

17

21–22. Exhaling, lower your trunk, raise your hips, and assume the triangular peak-like form shown in step 11. After repeating movements 7–14, bring your right foot forward. Next, bringing your left foot forward to the side of your right one,

18

assume the position shown in step 6. Repeating steps 5, 4, 3, and 2 in that order, finally assume the position in step 1.

19

20

21

22

Prostration Exercise

Goal and Effects

Both this and the preceding exercise promote mental unification. Though the prostration exercise is simpler, it is especially important in strengthening the legs and hips. Numerous repetitions of the same motions unify mind and body, regulate the breathing, and limber the body. Avoid tensing the little-toe side of the foot in this exercise, because it stiffens the neck and shoulders, stimulates the sympathetic nerves, and causes excitement. Concentrate on the big toes, hold the knees close together, and tense the abdomen. Bringing palms together in the prayerful attitude relaxes the shoulders and neck, corrects back and chest posture, and rectifies sagging of the rib cage. Tensing the big toes and standing on your toes improve your ability to maintain balance; lower the center of the body's weight; develop the legs, hips, and back; and promote the natural physical condition in which the upper part of the body is light and the lower part sound and heavy.

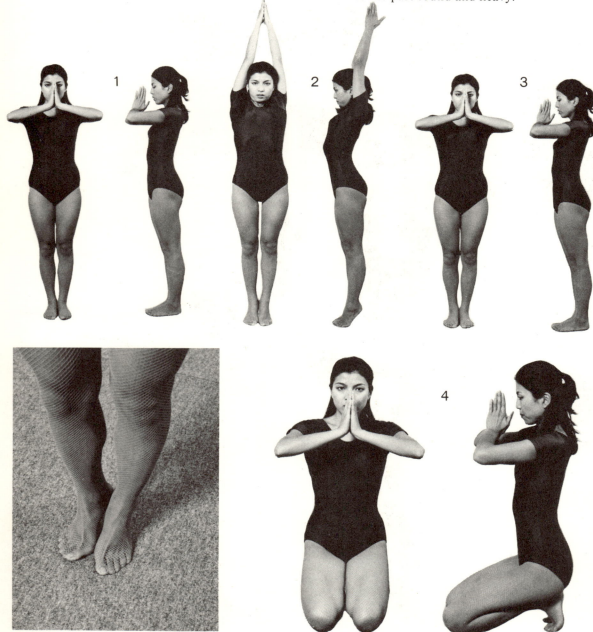

Emotionally, this exercise promotes a feeling of humility, penitence, and gratitude plus the willingness to be of service.

Movements and Breathing Order
1. With feet together and toes aligned, assume the prayerful position. The middle fingers of both hands must be tensed and must press together lightly at eye level. The elbows must be at shoulder level, and the forearms must form a straight, horizontal line. With chin pulled inward and neck and back extended, tense the insides of the knees and the thumbs and regulate your breathing.

Deliberately concentrate on the abdomen.
2. As you inhale, raise your hands—still palms together—high above your head. Your elbows must be extended straight, and your arms must touch your ears.
3. Gradually exhaling, return your arms to the positions they occupied in step 1.
4. As you inhale, rise on your toes. Then, exhaling, bend your knees and kneel until your buttocks rest on your heels.
5–6. Inhale. As you exhale, pull your toes inward until your insteps lie on the floor. You will be in the formal kneeling position known in Japanese as *seiza*. Your

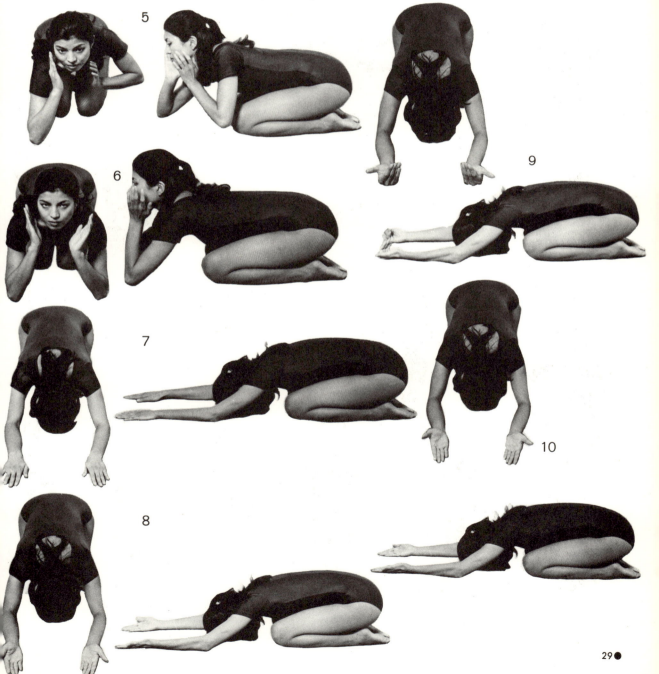

big toes should overlap. Inhaling, lean forward and extend your right elbow on the floor well in front of you. Then put your left elbow on the floor. Always begin with the right elbow. At the same time, thrust your chest well forward to extend your backbone. Thrusting your chest forward will bring your shoulders rearward and will slightly arch your back.

7.   As you exhale, put your forearms on the floor with palms down. At the same time, bring your forehead to the floor. Your buttocks must not leave your heels, and your abdomen and chest must lie along your thighs.

8–9.   With palms up and fingers bent slightly toward you, inhale.

10–11.   Returning your fingers to their original positions, once again turn palms downward and exhale.

12–13.   As you inhale, raise your trunk. Then bring first your left hand then your right hand toward your face into the prayer attitude.

14.   Turn your feet forward so that your body rests on your toes. Your buttocks should be resting on your heels.

15–16.   Tensing your big toes and inhaling, stand. Still inhaling, raise your hands as high above your head as you can.

17.   Exhaling, return to the position in step 1. Repeat at least one hundred and eight times.

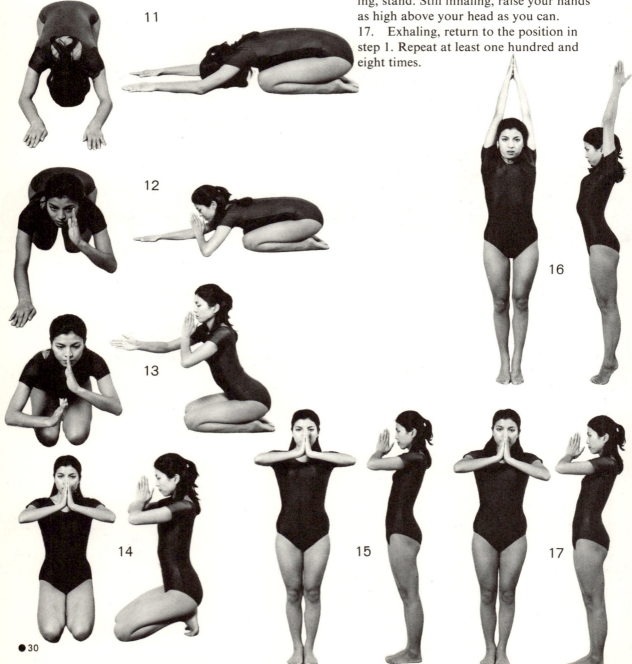

11

12

13

14

15

16

17

Self-diagnosis

Before you can solve the difficult problem of determining which of the Zen Yoga corrective exercises you need, you must diagnose yourself to discover abnormalities in your body. The exercises in this book are designed to correct conditions producing symptoms that are readily visible. The following charts and explanatory notes will assist you in diagnosing what is wrong and in selecting the exercises that can correct the trouble.

Basics
No matter whether you examine yourself in a mirror or have someone else examine you, observations must be made of your body in the following three positions.
1. *Standing:* Look for distortions and aberrations brought on by tension involved in the act of standing straight.
2. *Lying prone:* In this position, look for distortions and irregularities brought on by the total relaxation of this pose. In contrast to the stiffening occurring because of the tension of standing, the irregularities in this position will take the form of sagging and slackness.
3. *Kneeling in the formal* (seiza) *position:* This posture is midway between the tension of standing and the relaxation of lying prone.

Meaning of Diagnosis
Though diagnosis may be made on innumerable external and internal irregularities, this book concentrates on only some of the clearly apparent, external ones. In some cases, the aberration in surface areas—musculature—of the body affects internal organs. On the other hand, sometimes, the external disorder is only a protective reaction to the true cause of the trouble, which is to be found in the internal organs. In other words, some surface-level irregularities ought to be corrected, whereas others must not be treated, since they are only surface manifestations of internal disorders. For example, stiff shoulders are sometimes a manifestation of stomach disorder and sometimes indication that the muscles have stiffened in order to compensate for weakness in the skeleton. Thoughtlessly applied acupuncture, moxibustion, or shiatsu massage in an attempt to cure stiff shoulders brought on by internal disorders only aggravates the basic cause of the condition. In other words, diagnosis based on external visual examination only can lead to erroneous therapy. Though it is impossible to cover this complicated subject completely in the limits of a book like this one, I shall try to set forth the basics of self-diagnosis.

Many different elements can produce visible irregularities. For instance, when examination of a person lying down in the supine position shows that one leg is shorter than the other (p. 35), one of—or a combination of two or more of—the following may be causative factors: inclined pelvis, irregularities in the hip joint, imbalance in the abdominal muscles, irregularities in the internal organs, knee disorder, twisted neck, imbalance in the right or left ribs, imbalance in the right or left shoulder blade, arm irregularities, or twists in the hips.

It is very difficult to assign a cause to any single element and to treat that cause in the hope that it will relieve the condition. The situation is much more complicated, and the person performing therapy is ill-advised to treat, say, the arm simply because the arm is the location of the symptoms. Furthermore, the influence of the diet and of eating habits on bodily aberrations and irregularities is important. People who eat too much meat tend to have short left legs; and people who eat too many vegetables, short right legs.

Bearing the complicated nature of diagnosis in mind, examine yourself and use the corrective exercises that seem proper. If the desired effects are not forthcoming, seek further for the cause. Remember that the corrective exercises must bring about total therapy, must be general in effect, and must suit the individual patient and symptom.

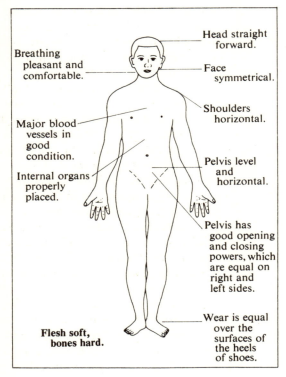

Head straight
forward.

Breathing
pleasant and
comfortable.

Face
symmetrical.

Shoulders
horizontal.

Major blood
vessels in
good
condition.

Internal organs
properly
placed.

Pelvis level
and
horizontal.

Pelvis has
good opening
and closing
powers, which
are equal on
right and
left sides.

Wear is equal
over the
surfaces of
the heels
of shoes.

**Flesh soft,
bones hard.**

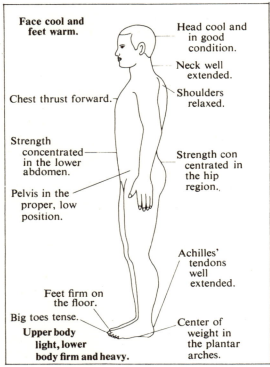

**Face cool and
feet warm.**

Head cool and
in good
condition.

Neck well
extended.

Chest thrust forward.

Shoulders
relaxed.

Strength
concentrated
in the lower
abdomen.

Strength con
centrated in
the hip
region.

Pelvis in the
proper, low
position.

Achilles'
tendons
well
extended.

Feet firm on
the floor.

Big toes tense.

**Upper body
light, lower
body firm and heavy.**

Center of
weight in
the plantar
arches.

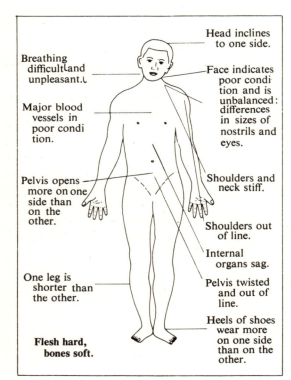

Head inclines
to one side.

Breathing
difficult and
unpleasant.

Face indicates
poor condi
tion and is
unbalanced:
differences
in sizes of
nostrils and
eyes.

Major blood
vessels in
poor condi
tion.

Shoulders and
neck stiff.

Pelvis opens
more on one
side than
on the
other.

Shoulders out
of line.

Internal
organs sag.

Pelvis twisted
and out of
line.

One leg is
shorter than
the other.

Heels of shoes
wear more
on one side
than on the
other.

**Flesh hard,
bones soft.**

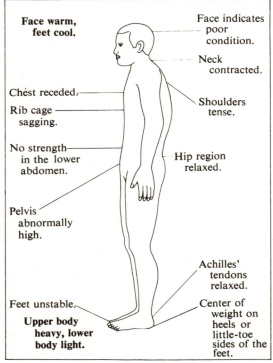

**Face warm,
feet cool.**

Face indicates
poor
condition.

Neck
contracted.

Chest receded.

Rib cage
sagging.

Shoulders
tense.

No strength
in the lower
abdomen.

Hip region
relaxed.

Pelvis
abnormally
high.

Feet unstable.

**Upper body
heavy, lower
body light.**

Achilles'
tendons
relaxed.

Center of
weight on
heels or
little-toe
sides of the
feet.

● Self-diagnosis 1

1. Head: The head and neck should be symmetrically arranged and should not lean in one direction. (A). Cases of extreme inclination (B) indicate that the muscles on the shortened side are contracted and stiff.

Causes and Related Parts
Twists on the right may mean irregularities in the right arm, right lung, liver, right side of the intestines, or right side of other internal organs. Often the right leg is shorter than the left; and the right ankle is stiff and weak.

Twists to the left indicate irregularities in the left arm, left lung, stomach twists to the left, abnormalities in the left hand, left lung, stomach, and left sides of such organs as the intestines.

Corrective Measures
Extend the short and stiff leg to limber the ankle. Perform exercises to tense and strengthen the opposite leg.

2. Shoulders: The shoulders should be straight, on the same level, and of the same height. They should not incline to one side, forward, or rearward. Correct, normal shoulders and shoulder positions are shown in A, C, and E. In B, the right shoulder sags and is wider than the left. In D, the shoulders are pulled abnormally forward.

Causes and Related Parts
When the chest is weak and both shoulders are pulled forward, the buttocks are weak, the lungs are weak, and the person is probably highly susceptible to colds.

Corrective Measures
Employ exercises that strengthen and pull the buttocks rearward.

Weak and retracted hips (plus weak knees) indicate irregularities in the reproductive, urinary, and digestive organs or aging (abdominal irregularities).

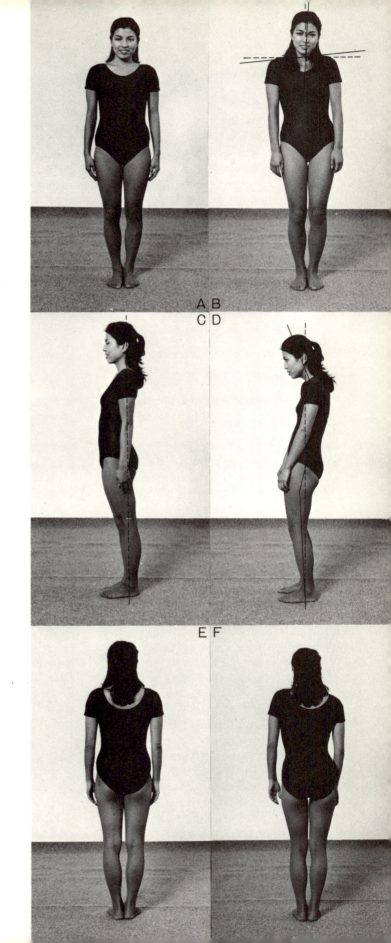

A B
C D

E F

Corrective Measures

Employ exercises that call for bending the hips rearward and for moving the body in various directions.

Straight shoulders and forward inclined neck indicate slackness in the cranium caused by too little or too much sleep, stiffness in the hips, incomplete evacuation of body wastes, or overeating.

Corrective Measures

Employ exercises that call for great backward bending pulling the chin inward, extending the neck, and lifting the cranium.

Shoulders pulled too far to the rear indicate slackness in the digestive or reproductive systems.

Corrective Measures

Employ exercises calling for forward leaning and for tensing of the feet only.

When the left shoulder only is pulled too far forward, hardening of the arteries, coronary ailments, and chilling are indicated.

When the right shoulder only is pulled too far forward, circulation is incomplete; and the liver may be out of order.

When both shoulders are pulled upward too far, the neck is stiff and tense, the brain tires easily, and the organs of perception are out of order.

When only one shoulder droops, there is usually an organic abnormality on the side of the drooping.

Corrective Measures

Employ exercises that call for strong twisting and leaning to the right and left and that raise the sagging shoulder or force the high shoulder to lower.

3. Chest Region: Normarlly, right-left symmetry is maintained, the chest is wide, and the nipples of the breats are pointed forward. Pay attention to the positions of the nipples and breasts, difference in chest width on the right and left, expanse and angles of the lower ribs, contraction of the chest muscles, and relative softness of the abdomen.

Causes of Trouble and Related Parts

Irregularities in the height of the upper part of the chest indicate trouble with the respiratory organs and the heart.

When the right side of the chest is wider and higher than the left, liver trouble is indicated. When the left side is wider and higher, stomach trouble is likely.

Too acute an angle in the lowest ribs indicates weak respiratory organs and general sagging of the ribs and internal organs.

4. Abdominal Region: Criteria of judgment include the right and left widths of the abdomen, differences in elevation of the abdomen on the right and left, position of the navel, and relative hardness or softness to the touch. The navel should be in the center; the entire region should be suitably elastic; and the abdomen should be retracted. A protruding abdomen indicates slackness.

Causes and Related Parts

Stiffness above the diaphragm indicates abnormalities above the neck, nervous tension, and unbalance in the autonomous nervous system. Tension on one side of the trunk indicates abnormalities in the hand and inter nal organs on the same side.

Displacement of the navel in any direction indicates displacement of the internal organs in the same direction. Abnormal height of the navel indicates abnormalities of the internal organs on the side on which the navel is higher. When the long bone is higher on one side, the body is twisted. When it is longer on one side, the body inclines in the direction of the longer part.

Forward projection of the pubic bone indicates forward inclination of the pelvis. Excessive recession of the pubic bone indicates rearward inclination of the pelvis.

5. Examining the hands and arms: Too long arms are caused by slackness in the shoulders; too short arms are caused by stiff shoulders.

Lack of extendability in the elbows indicates disorders in the hips and the internal organs.

Discrepancies in the twists of the right and left hands indicate imbalance in the right and left ribs and abnormal placement of the shoulder blades.

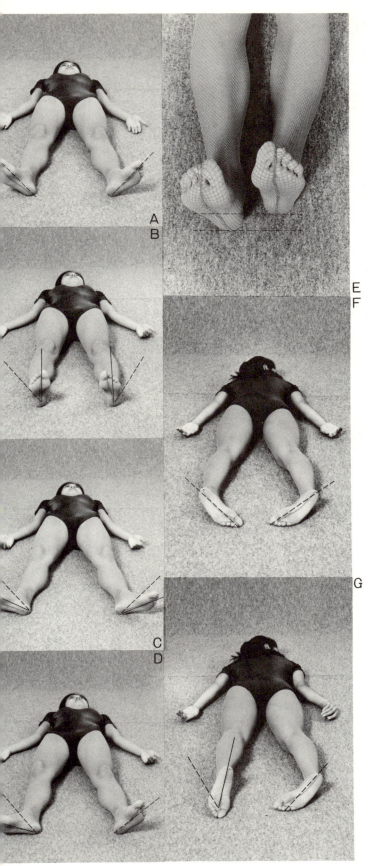

6. *Leg and Foot Region:* Normally, the legs should be the same length, symmetrical, and open to an angle of roughly sixty degrees (A).

Causes of Trouble and Related Parts
When the legs are too close in the supine position (B), the pelvis is constantly closed; and there may be irregularities in the neck and chest.

When the legs are too far apart in the supine position (C), the pelvis is constantly open; and there may be irregularities in the abdominal organs.

When one leg falls much farther open than the other (D), organs on that side may be slack or anemia may have set in. Constant muscular contraction and blood congestion may be the cause of the failure of one leg to fall open as far as the other. Touching will show that the leg that has fallen too far open is slack, whereas the other one is tense. When the person stands, the slack leg will become contracted and rigid.

Discrepancies in leg length (E) indicate pelvic inclination and internal organic irregularities on the side of the short leg.

In the prone position, the feet and legs assume the position in (G) if they are normal. The foot position in (G) indicates organic irregularities and twisting of the pelvis.

7. *Back Region:* Points to be investigated in diagnosis from this angle are as follows. Does the back appear symmetrical right and left? Is the backbone straight? Are the vertebrae equally spaced? Do any of them protrude? If so, which ones? Are the shoulder blades symmetrically placed right and left and up and down? Are the buttocks resilient and strong?

Causes of Trouble and Related Parts
If the back rises higher on one side than the other, there is trouble in the internal organs on that side; and the backbone may be twisted.

Though the symptoms vary with the part affected, curvature, protrusions, and overly close placement of the vertebrae indicate pressure on the nervous system and total physical disorder. Slackness on one side or the other of the buttocks indicates trouble in the intestines or reproductive organs on that side.

8. *Examination from the Kneeling Position:* In the correct kneeling position, the shoulders form a horizontal line intersecting at right angles with lines dropped from the top of the head vertically through the ears, the point of the shoulders, and the hips.

Causes of Trouble and Related Parts
In the posture in (B), it is clearly noticed that the shoulders, the neck and the hips are out of order.

In the posture in (C), the left shoulder droops, the right hip is twisted inward, the left hip is twisted outward, the spine

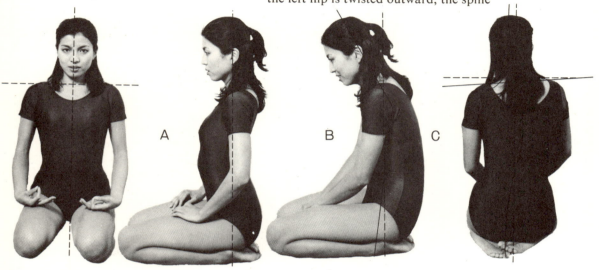

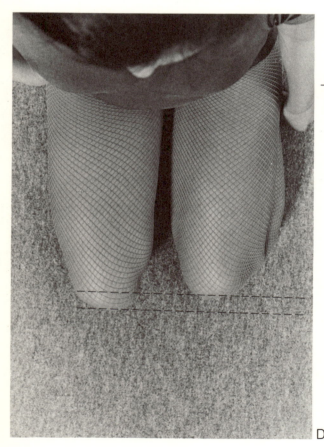

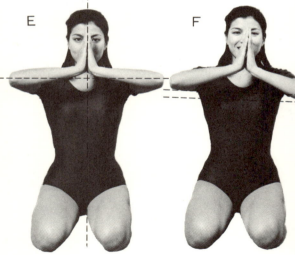

curves to the right, and the vertebrae incline to the right. This posture will cause pain in the right hip and the area below the left shoulder blade.

In the position in (D), the lower part of the body is twisted to the left; and one knee projects beyond the other.

(E) shows the correct prayerful-hands position. In (F), the left elbow is too low; and the shoulders, neck, and shoulder blades are abnormal.

●Self-diagnosis 2

Discovering and correcting irregularities by means of basic poses and motions.

1.   Supine position, with arms extended forward: Have someone check arm lengths and the contraction of the muscles of the shoulder blades (A).

Corrective Measures

Have your assistant sit beside you on the side of the shorter arm. The assistant supports the hand of that arm in one hand and presses on the lower edge of the shoulder blade with the other. Exhaling, twist the shorter arm inward and outward as you extend it. The assistant must move upward on the muscles around the shoulder blade (B).

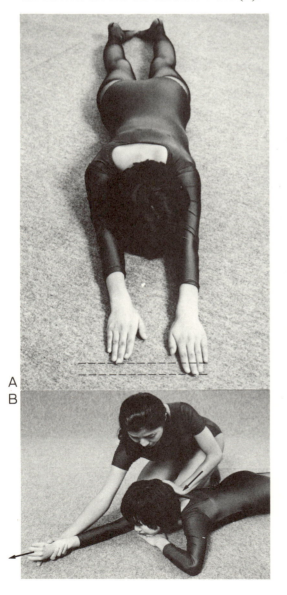

A
B

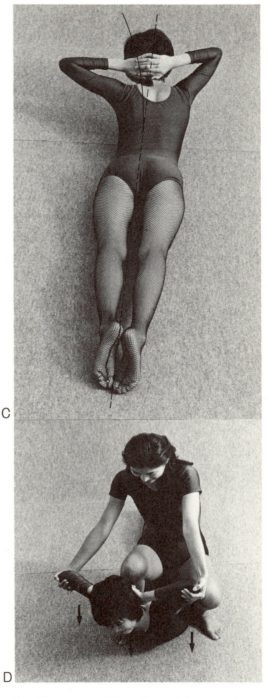

C

D

2.   Curvature of the spine: Lie on your stomach with your hands locked behind your head and with your elbows extended to the sides (C). The model's spine curves leftward. The muscles on the left are contracted more than the ones on the right, causing the spine and entire upper body to bend to the left.·

Corrective Measures

The assistant must sit on your buttocks and press one knee lightly against the spine. While the assistant attempts to raise and bend your upper body in the direction opposite that of the abnormal curvature (in this case, to the right), exhale and exert all of your strength to press your body against the floor. Tense fully then, suddenly exhaling, relax entirely.

3.   *Twists in the hips and right or left bends in the legs:*   When you lie prone on the floor, with legs positioned naturally, your feet would assume the positions shown in (F) on p. 35. In this case (A), however, the right leg is turned inward, indicating twist in the hips and a bend in the leg.

Corrective Measures

The assistant turns your right foot outward and your left foot inward (B) and presses lightly on your heels with both

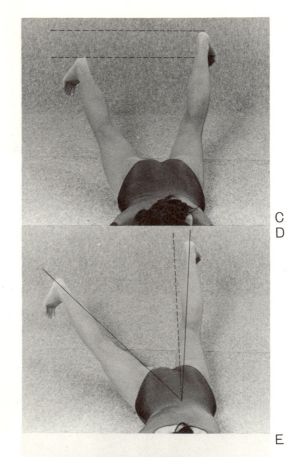

C
D

E

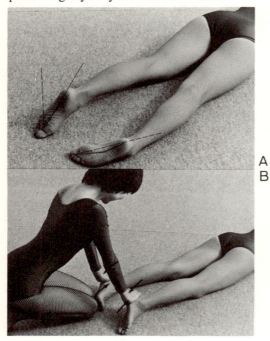

A
B

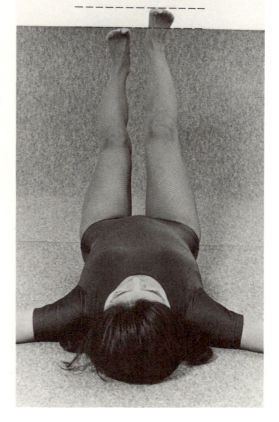

hands. As you exhale, attempt to return your feet to the positions they occupied in (A). The assistant holds them at the point where the heels are turned directly upward for a few seconds then lets them go, as you exhale suddenly and relax. (Gradually it will become easy to do this on the side on which it was difficult.)

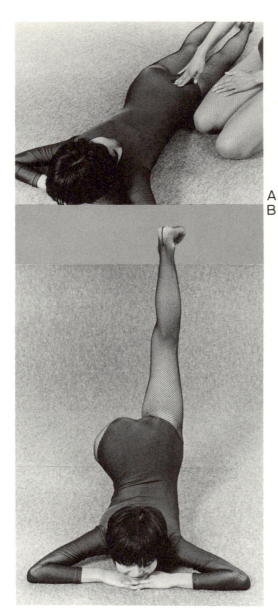

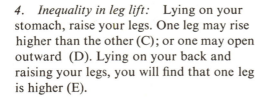

A
B

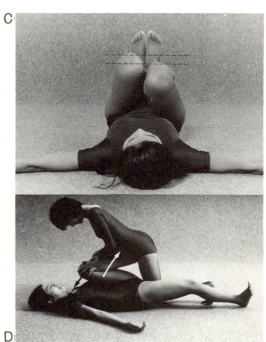

C

D

5. Discrepancies in leg bend: Lying on your back, draw your knees up.

Corrective Measures
Draw the affected leg upward and have the assistant press on that knee toward your chest as you resist the action (D).

6. Have your assistant check the height of your buttocks: In A, the right buttock is high.

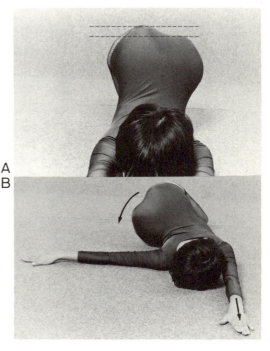

A
B

4. Inequality in leg lift: Lying on your stomach, raise your legs. One leg may rise higher than the other (C); or one may open outward (D). Lying on your back and raising your legs, you will find that one leg is higher (E).

Corrective Measures
Equalize the lift and spread of your legs. Have the assistant press to discover which buttock is less firm. With your hands together under your chin and your knees on the floor (B), lift the leg on the affected side several times to firm the buttock.

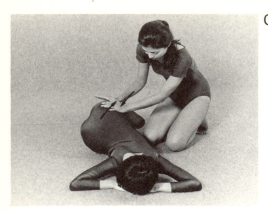

C

7. Bends in the neck:

Bends in the neck: Assuming the cobra pose—*Bhujangasana*—(flat on your stomach with the upper part of your body from the chest raised and with hands flat on the floor by your side; A), have the assistant check your neck for straightness. In the photograph, the model's neck is twisted to the right.

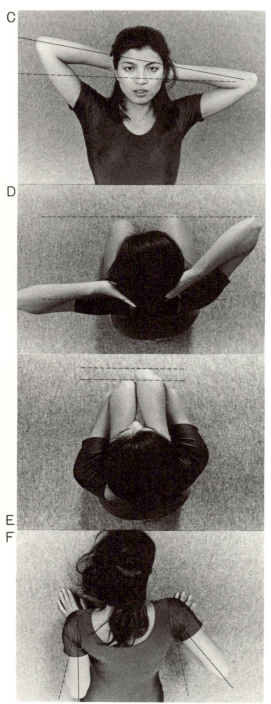

Corrective Measures

Stretch the arm affected directly to the side and role your hips in that direction (B). When you are working with someone, have that person press on the buttock that is too low as you resist and raise it.

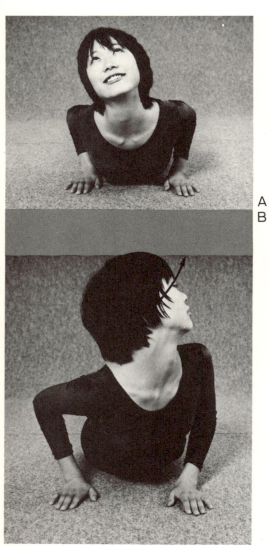

Corrective Measures

Turn your neck and head several times in the direction opposite to that of the twist.

8. *Inequalities in elbow placement:* Kneeling, place your hands behind your head and extend your bent arms to the side. The photographs (C and D) show

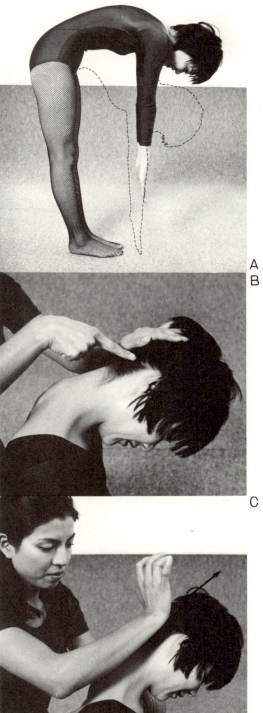

A
B

C

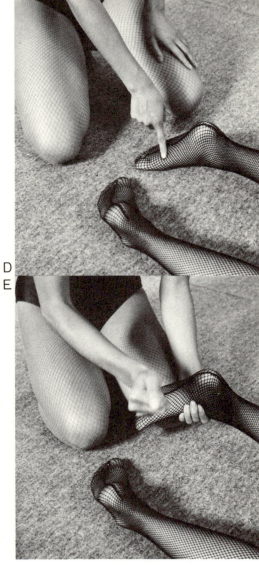

D
E

inequalities of height and projection: the right elbow is higher and advanced farther forward than the left one.

Corrective Measures

Throughout all the exercises in this book, make a deliberate effort to equalize elbow heights and projections. When the elbows are pulled forward (E), one will project beyond the other. When you lie on your stomach, with hands on the floor under your arms, your shoulder blades will be out of line.

9. *Forward bending pose (Paschimotka-sana):*   Abnormalities in the upper and lower part of the hip region revealed when you are unable to touch your toes (A).

Corrective Measures

Contraction in the back of the neck is related to this condition. To correct it, have your assistant tap from top to bottom about ten times on the hollow in the nape of your neck (B–C). In addition, have your assistant tap the arch of the foot at the base of the big toe, a place that is related to the lumbar vertebrae (D–E).

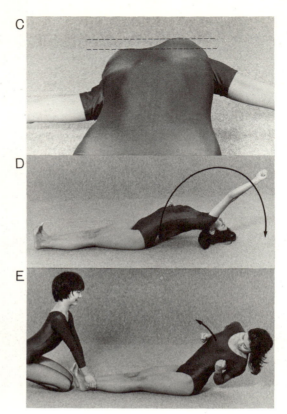

C

D

E

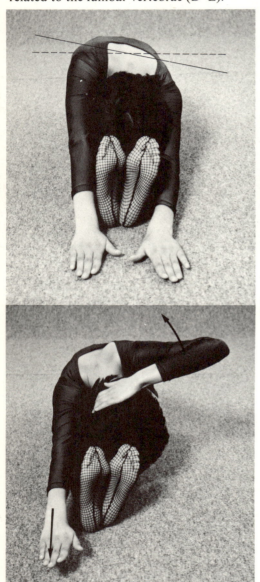

A
B

and, inhaling and exhaling, attempt to bring the right side of our chest as close to your leg as possible.

11. *Chest height discrepancies revealed in the fish pose (Matsyasana):* In the photograph, the left side is high (C).

10. *Discrepancies in back level revealed in the forward bending pose:* The right side of the model's back is higher than the left (A).

Corrective Measures

Stretching your right hand forward and holding the back of your head with your left hand (B), lower your left shoulder

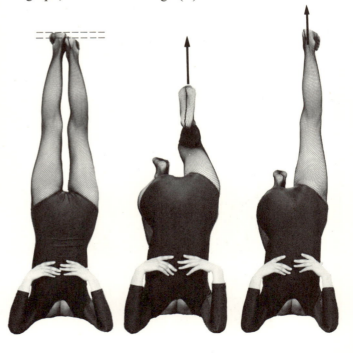

Corrective Measures

Extend and raise and lower the side on which the chest is higher (D). When you are working with someone, have that person hold your ankles while you thrust the lower side of your chest forward and upward (E). Repeat several times.

12.   Shoulder standing pose (Sarvanga-sana): In the photograph, the model's left leg is shorter (A).

Corrective Measures

Retract both legs as you inhale. Exhaling, kick the shorter leg straight upward, keeping the Achilles' tendon extended all the time (B–C). Repeat.

13.   Inability to extend the upper back and neck fully revealed in the shoulder-stand position: Your legs and hips should be directly above your shoulders. The photograph (A) indicates inability to extend the neck and upper back fully.

Corrective Measures

Lie on your stomach and have the assistant press the underside of one foot against the toes of one of your feet and, gripping the ankle of that same foot with both hands, pull to extend the Achilles' tendon (B). Repeat with the other foot. Inability to extend the Achilles' tendon fully prevents your being able to extend your neck fully and thus makes the perfect shoulder stand impossible.

14.   Flexibility of the pelvic joint revealed in the kneeling position with the soles of the feet together: The knees should touch the floor. In this case (C), the hips are

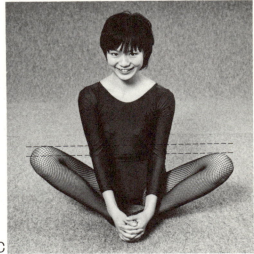

C

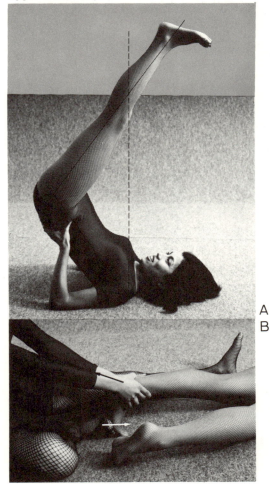

A
B

D

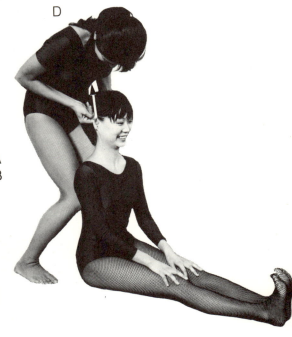

43 ●

tilted rearward; and the knees are off the floor at unequal heights.

Corrective Measures

As you sit comfortably on the floor (D), the assistant grips the upper parts of your ears and pulls upward. This will make it easier for you to put your knees on the floor.

15. *Side muscular contraction and pelvic displacement revealed in the fish-hook pose* (*Trikonasana*): Executing the fish-hook pose, bend first to the right side then to the left. The model finds it hard to bend to the right (A–B).

Corrective Measures

Lock your hands behind your head and bend in the direction in which bending is difficult. Have your assistant grip your elbows and pull you in that direction as you exhale and exert as much power as possible to raise your body in the opposite direction. Hold the pose for a few seconds and then suddenly relax (C).

16. *Discovering muscular, skeletal, and*

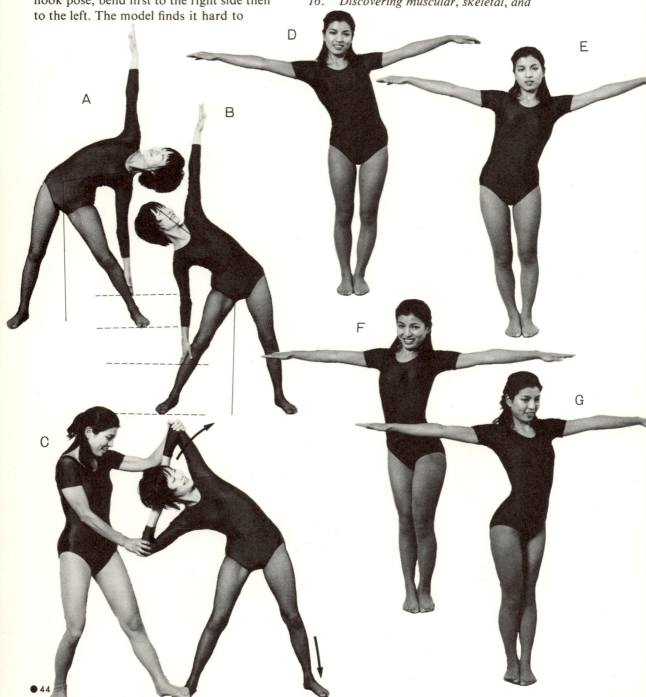

organic irregularities by swinging your hips (D–G).

Corrective Measures
Always make a deliberate effort to repeat all difficult positions and movements as often as you can.

17.   Difficulties in raising the legs in the bow pose (Dhanurasana):
In the photograph, the model experiences difficulty in raising her left leg.

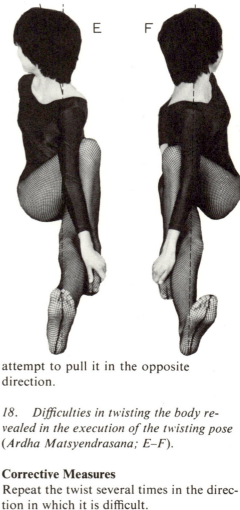

Corrective Measures
When working alone, pull the leg that is difficult to lift upward with both hands (B–C). When working with someone, have your assistant grip and pull the leg as you grip it with both hands and

attempt to pull it in the opposite direction.

18.   Difficulties in twisting the body revealed in the execution of the twisting pose (Ardha Matsyendrasana; E–F).

Corrective Measures
Repeat the twist several times in the direction in which it is difficult.

19.1   Hip-height discrepancies revealed in the plow pose (Halasana) (A).

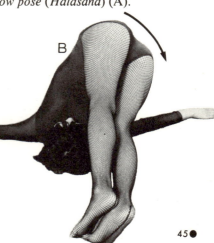

Corrective Measures

Turn several times in the direction in which the hip is higher (B).

19.2 Leg-length discrepancies in the same pose (C).

Corrective Measures

Bending the long leg, extend the Achilles' tendon of the short one several times (D).

19.3 Arm-length discrepancies.

Corrective Measures

Extend the longer arm over your head. Leaving the short arm in place, extend and contract your knees (F).

20. The arch pose—Shyakulasana—used to reveal lack of extendibility from the shoulder to the arm: In the photograph (A), the right arm lacks extendibility.

Corrective Measures

The assistant twists and pulls the arm that will not rise easily, as you resist this movement and attempt to return the hand to

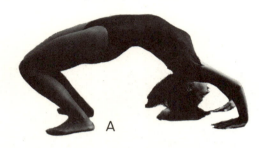

its original position. When a maximum of force is being generated, suddenly exhale and relax. Repeat several times, having the assistant gradually lower the arm to the side.

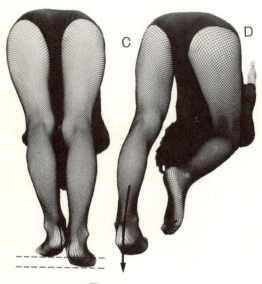

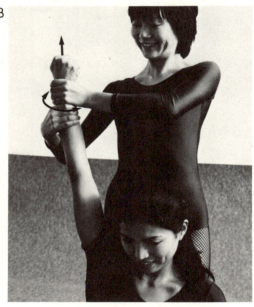

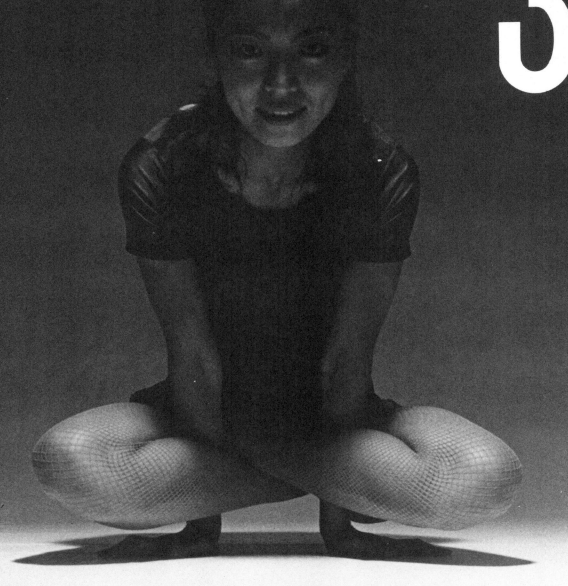

Heaviness and Aching in the Head

These exercises are intended to bring relief from headaches caused by something other than actual illness of the brain. Stiffening in the shoulders and sagging of the cranium are the most frequent causes. Distortions in the body and irregularities in the related organs cause aching on one side of the head. The direct cause of the pain or heaviness is tension of the brain blood vessels, which, in turn, is caused by incorrect posture, stercoral incarceration, organic, abnormalities, emotional upsets, and incorrect diet. The exercises below correct stiffening in the shoulders and sagging of the cranial bones. The following relations exist between various parts of the head and the internal organs: the front part is related to the stomach, the liver, and the heart; the top, to the anus and reproductive organs; the sides to the intestines; and the rear, to the kidneys.

Movements and Breathing Order
1. Kneeling in the *seiza* position, inhale and lift and tense your shoulders.
2. Abruptly exhale as you relax your shoulders and neck and allow your head to drop. Repeat.

Effects
Tensing and abruptly relaxing the neck and shoulders relieve blood congestion in those areas and improve circulation in the brain.

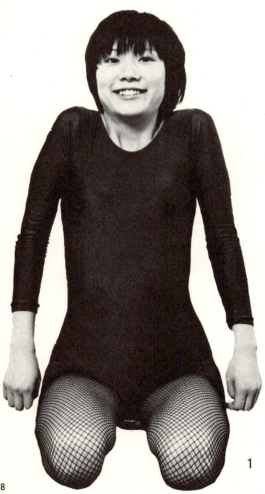

1

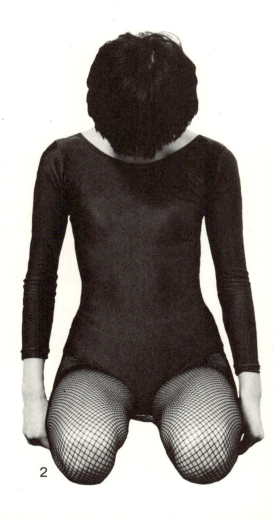

2

Movements and Breathing Order

1. Kneeling in the *seiza* position, join your hands behind your back and extend your neck upward as far as you can.
2. As you exhale, stretching your neck, bend your head forward and backward, right and left, making a complete turn (A–F). Each time your head returns to the central position, inhale. Perform these head bends slowly, remaining aware of the extension of the neck. Make use of the weight of the head.

Effects

This exercise corrects the placement of the shoulder blades, relieves blood congestion, limbers the muscles, and rests the head.

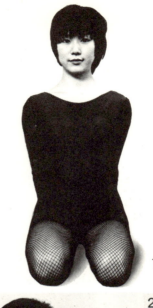

1

2– A 2– C   2– E

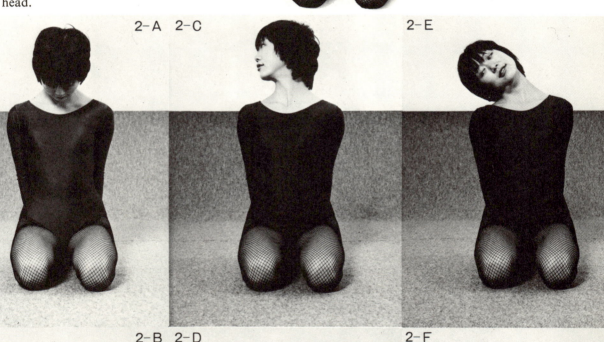

2– B 2– D   2– F

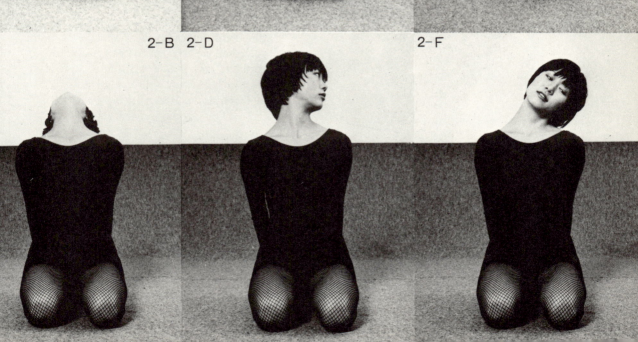

Movements and Breathing Order

1–2. As you exhale, press both hands to the front and back, then right and left, of the skull. Press more often in the direction in which pressure feels good.

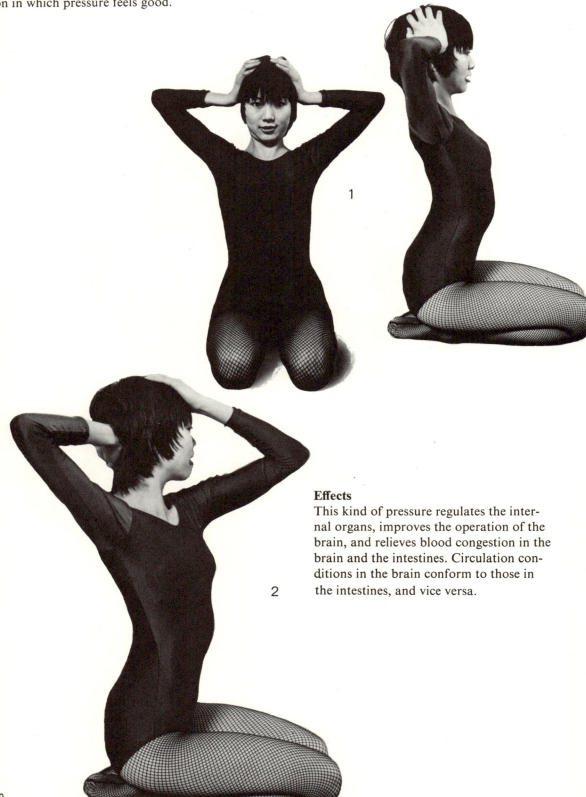

1

2

Effects

This kind of pressure regulates the internal organs, improves the operation of the brain, and relieves blood congestion in the brain and the intestines. Circulation conditions in the brain conform to those in the intestines, and vice versa.

Movements and Breathing Order

1–2.   Feel the base of the head to determine the direction in which the cranium sags. Then lightly tap on this side, from bottom upward, with your fist. Have your assistant examine your head from behind; the side on which the ear is lower is the sagging one.

Effects

Tapping corrects the position of the cranium and relieves blood congestion in the brain.

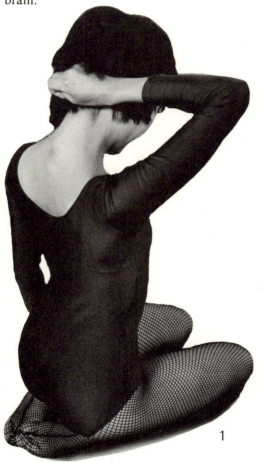

1

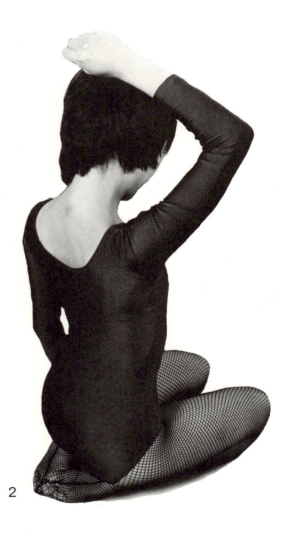

2

Movements and Breathing Order

Kneel in the *seiza* position. Have your assistant press on the back, the left back, and the right back of your head. Inhale and, as you exhale, press your head in resistance against the assistant's hands (A, B, and C). Repeat more often in the directions in which the pressure feels good.

Effects

This exercise corrects the position of the back of the head, rests the neck muscles, and improves circulation in them.

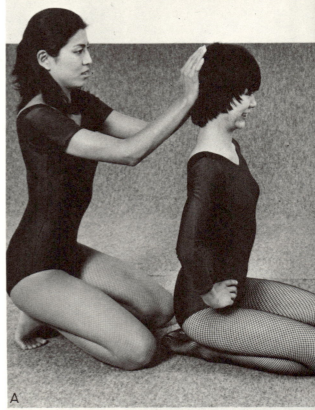

A

B C

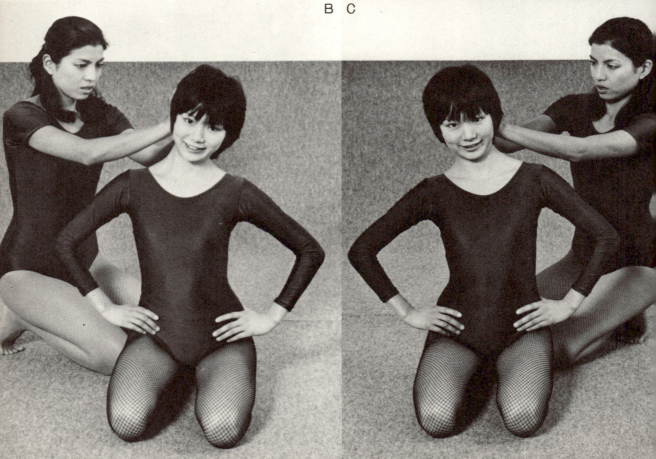

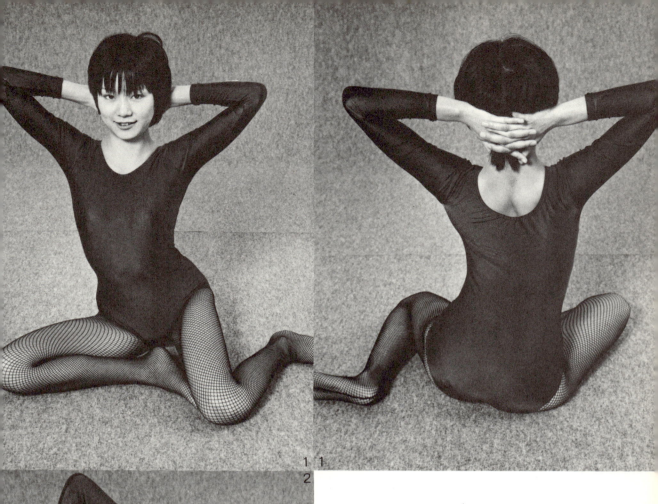
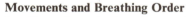

Movements and Breathing Order

1.   From the *seiza* kneeling position, lower one buttock to the floor and bend the leg on that side outward. Lock your hands behind your head.

2.   Inhale and, as you exhale, with one hand raise the back of one side of your head and bend your body in the same direction. Inhale as you return your body upright. Repeat. Perform this exercise more often in the direction in which it is difficult.

Effects

Bending relieves blood congestion in the abdomen and improves circulation. Raising one side of the rear of the head corrects the placement of the cranium and relieves blood congestion.

Movements and Breathing Order

Lying on your back with your hands behind your head, inhale and, as you exhale, pull your head as if it were a cork you were trying to pull from a bottle. Keep your Achilles' tendons tensed. Pull first one side then the other, then both at once. Pull harder on the side that sags and repeat several times.

Effects

This exercise corrects the placement of the cranium and firms the head while correcting looseness in the intestines.

Movements and Breathing Order ▶

1. Lying on your back, bend your knees and bring both hands together on your chest in the prayerful attitude.
2. Inhaling and exhaling, raise your hips and shoulders till your body is supported by your feet and head only. Take a deep breath and hold the pose.

Effects

Putting your weight on your head in this way stimulates and relieves blood congestion in the head and neck. Raising your shoulders and hips corrects faults in the spinal column.

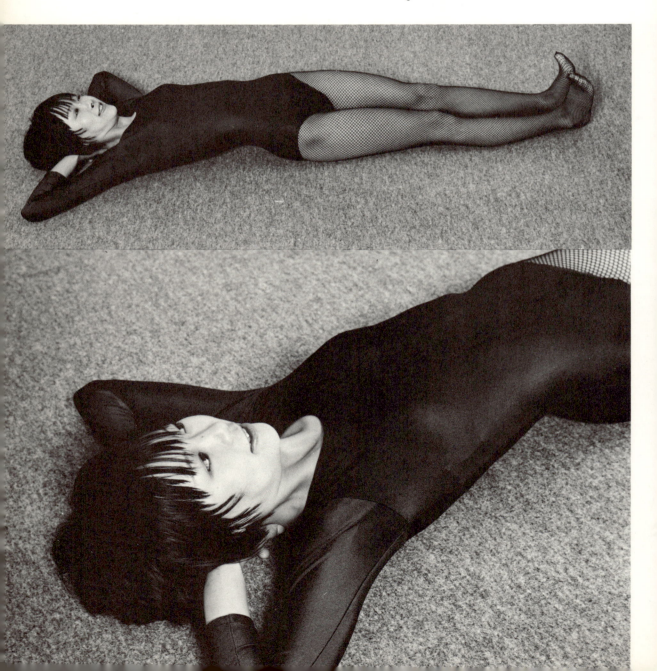

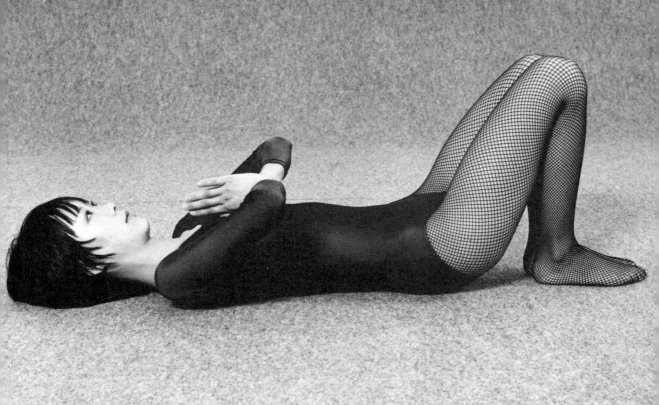

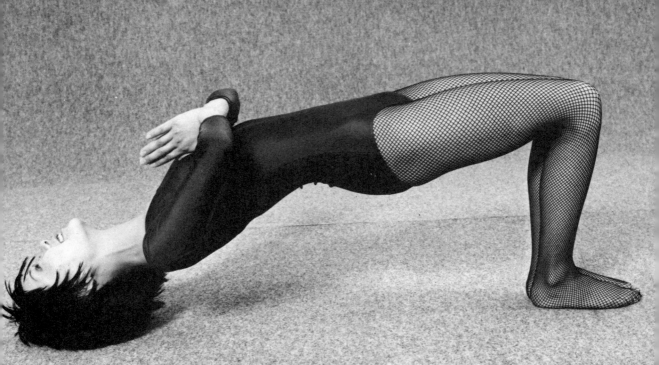

Movements and Breathing Order

1. Lying on your stomach, put only the toes of your feet on the floor and spread your feet about as far apart as your shoulders are wide. Lock your fingers behind your head and extend your elbows straight to the sides.

2. Inhale and, as you exhale, press one side of your head upward with one hand and bend your trunk in the same direction. Inhaling, return your trunk to the normal position; then, exhaling, bend in the opposite direction. Repeat more often on the side on which the cranium sags.

Effects

This corrects sagging of the cranium, relieves contraction in the chest, and eliminates blood congestion in the lumbar vertebrae. Furthermore, it strengthens the back and thus make it easier for you to maintain good posture.

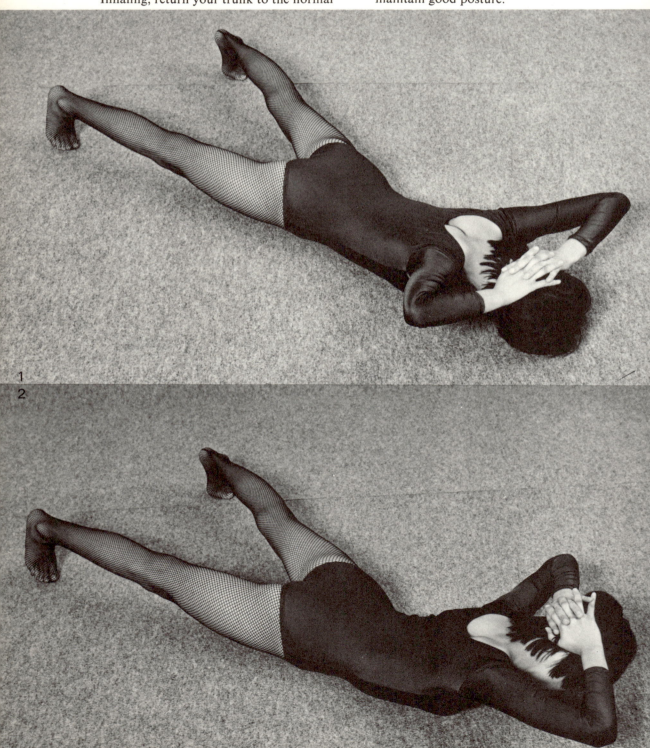

Movements and Breathing Order

1. Lying on your stomach, bend one leg outward, lock your fingers behind your head, and extend your elbows to the sides.

2. Inhale, then exhaling, raise one side of your head with one hand and bend your trunk in the same direction. At this time, strongly extend the Achilles' tendon of the straight leg. Inhaling, return your trunk to the central position. Straightening the bent leg and bending the other, repeat in the opposite direction. Repeat more times in the direction of the side on which the cranium sags.

Effects

Bending the body relieves contraction in the opposite half, and relieves blood congestion in the head and upper body. It also corrects irregularities in the pelvis.

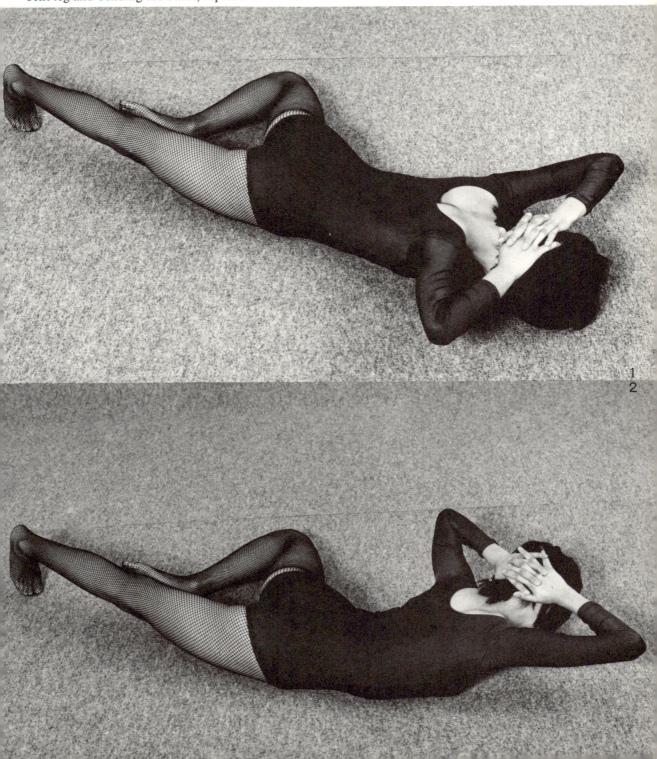

1
2

Insomnia

Goals and Effects

Total insomnia is impossible. What usually goes under the name *insomnia* is partial lack of slumber or shallow sleep. Relaxation of the new and old cortexes of the cerebrum brings about sleep. Stimulation of them prevents sleep. Such stimulation can arise from physical or mental causes. The old cortex, which controls desires, instincts, and emotions, is related to the internal organs. Emotional upset or organic disorders stimulate it and prevent sleep. Some of the physical causes of such stimulation include constipation or accumulation of urine in the bladder, undigested food in the stomach, stiff muscles, localized fatigue, and poor circulation. To induce sleep, the muscles must relax, the breathing must be calm, and the parasympathetic nervous system must be in control of the body. These exercises are intended to relax tension in the shoulders, neck, upper body, chest, and abdomen and to loosen the pelvis.

Movements and Breathing Order

1. Lying on your back, put both elbows on the floor and spread your feet (Achilles' tendons tensed) to about the width of your hips.
2. Inhaling, tense and raise your hips from the floor.
3. Abruptly relax and allow your body to fall to the floor. At the same time exhale. Repeat.

Effects

This exercise limbers the hips and the pelvis. Limbering the pelvis has a softening effect on the entire body.

1

2
3

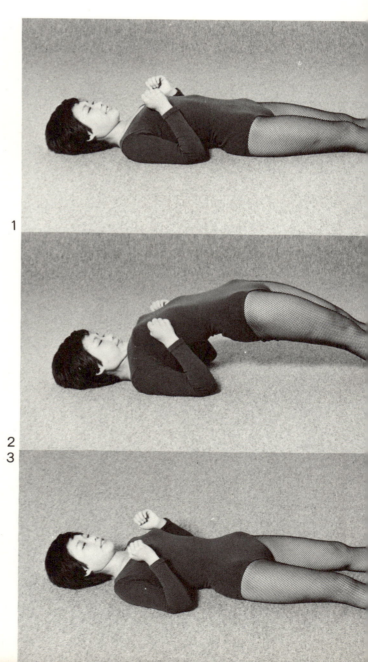

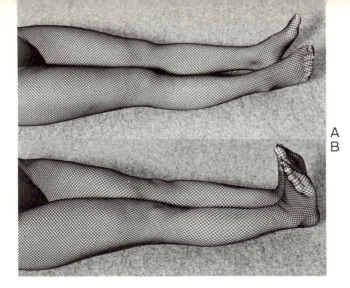

A
B

Movements and Breathing Order

1. Lying on your back, extend your arms to the side and tense both Achilles' tendons.

2. Inhaling and exhaling, turn both hands inward then outward as you further tense your neck and your Achilles' tendons. Abruptly relax. Repeat. The Achilles' tendons can best be tensed if the heels are raised slightly from the floor (A and B).

Effects

This corrects elevation of the body's center of balance caused by contraction of the Achilles' tendons and fatigue in the head.

1
2

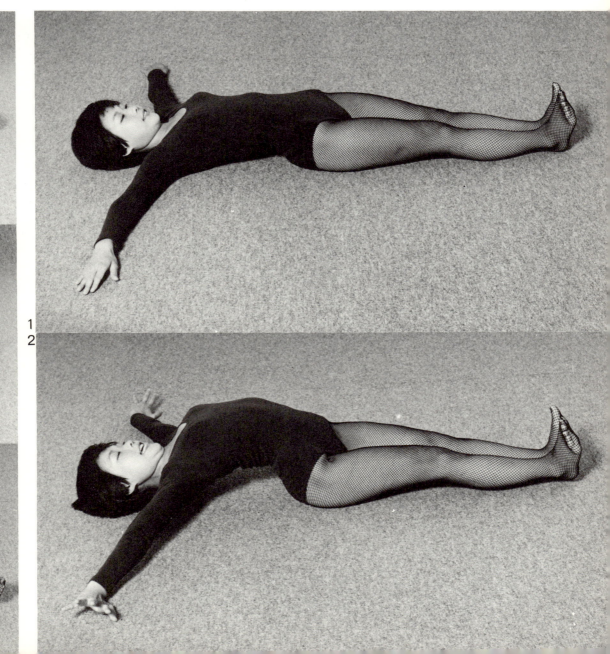

Movements and Breathing Order

1. Lying on our back, with legs and feet together, lock your hands behind your head and extend your elbows to the sides.

2. Inhale and, as you exhale, strongly tense your Achilles' tendons. At the same time, pull the back of your neck as if your head were a cork you were pulling from a bottle. Extend your elbows and neck. Suddenly relax. Repeat.

Effects

This corrects elevation of the body's center of balance caused by contraction of the Achilles' tendons and fatigue in the head. Furthermore, it corrects sagging of the back part of the head and, by pulling the scalp, improves circulation.

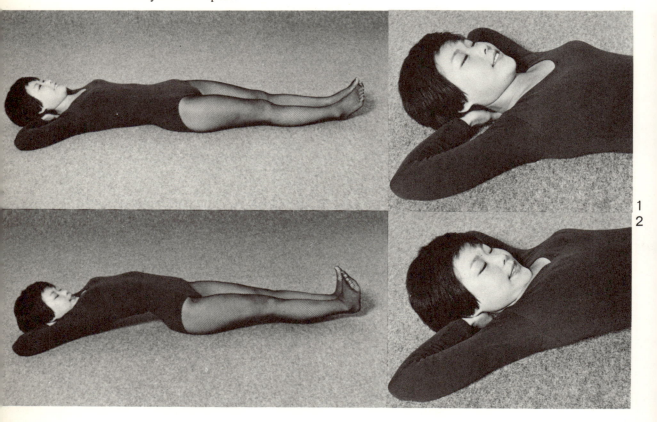

1
2

Movements and Breathing Order

1. Lying on your back, bring both legs together and lock your hands behind your head.
2. Inhaling and exhaling, extend your Achilles' tendon. At the same time, gripping the back of your head with both hands, pull your head upward until your chin reaches your chest. Abruptly relax and return to the position in step 1.

Effects

In addition to the effects produced by the preceding exercise, this one corrects abnormalities in the cervical vertebrae.

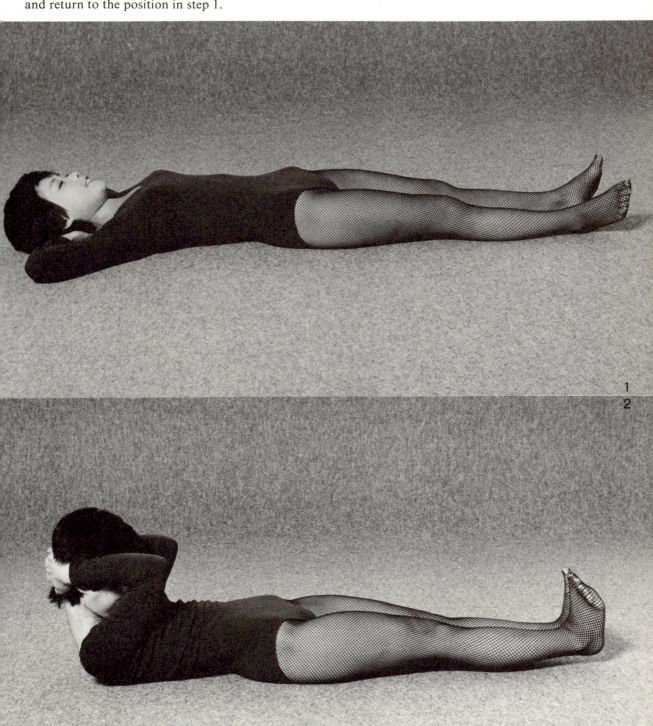

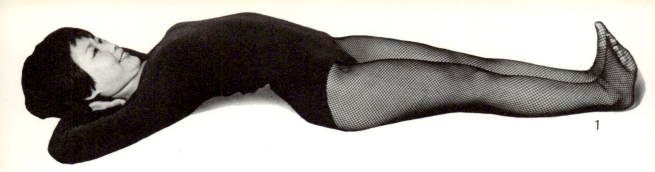

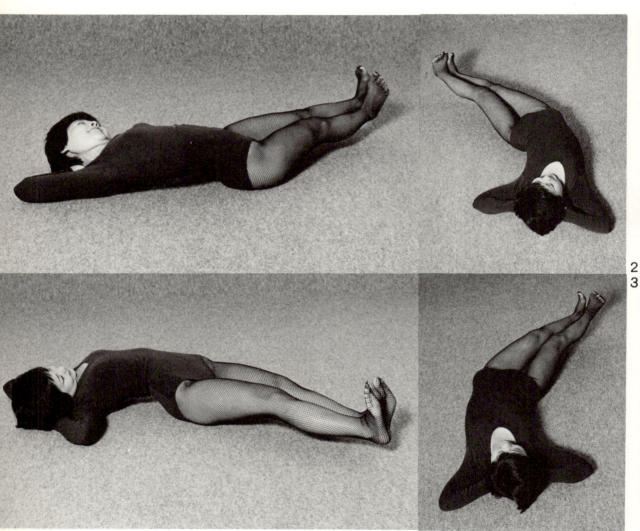

Movements and Breathing Order

1. Lying on your back with your hands locked behind your head and your elbows extended, bring both legs together, extend your Achilles' tendons, and raise your feet off the floor.

2. Inhale then, as you exhale, press on the right side of the rear of your head with your right hand. Slide the right elbow in the direction of your head and swing both legs to the left.

3. Inhaling, return to the position in step 1. Exhaling, swing to the right. Repeat several times. This exercise is more effective if, at its conclusion, you raise your feet thirty centimeters off the floor as you inhale and lower them to five centimeters from the floor as you exhale.

Effects

This improves circulation in the head by pulling the scalp and improves respiration.

Movements and Breathing Order

1. Lying on your back, relax. Bring your hands upward toward your armpits, extend your elbows to the sides, and extend your legs.

2. Inhaling, then exhaling, bring your legs as close together as possible and extend your Achilles' tendons. Without taking them off the floor, slide your elbows as far upward as possible. Raise your feet about five centimeters from the floor. Holding this position, breathe slowly for a while. Suddenly relax and allow your body to fall back to the floor.

Effects

This exercise cures elevation of the body's center of balance and weakness in the chest and upper back resulting from lack of strength in the abdomen.

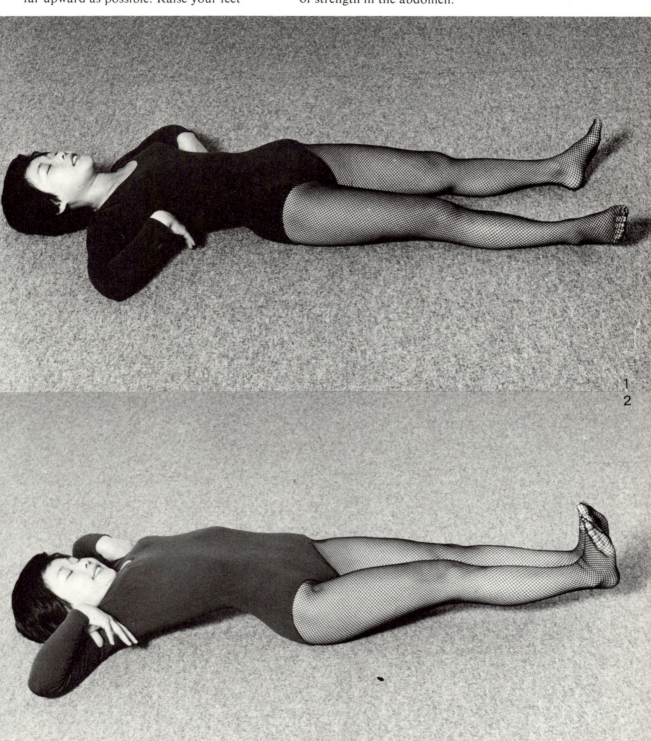

1
2

Movements and Breathing Order

1. Lying on your back, bring your hands upward toward your armpits. Bring your legs together, extend your Achilles' tendons, and raise your feet five centimeters from the floor.

2. As you inhale and exhale, leaving it on the floor, slide your right elbow upward as if you were shrugging that shoulder. At the same time, slide both feet to the left.

3. Inhale as you bring your legs to the central position again. Then repeat the exercise in the opposite direction. Repeat.

Effects

This exercise improves circulation in the head by relieving stiffness in the neck and shoulders. Furthermore, it strengthens the abdomen and lowers the body's center of balance.

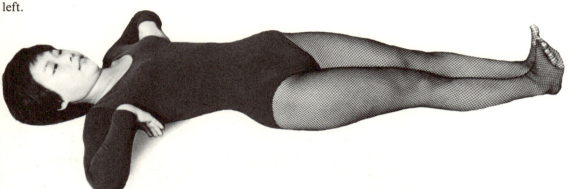

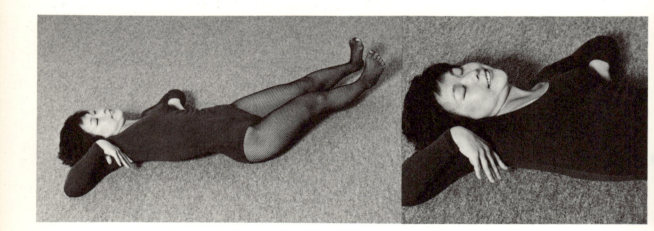

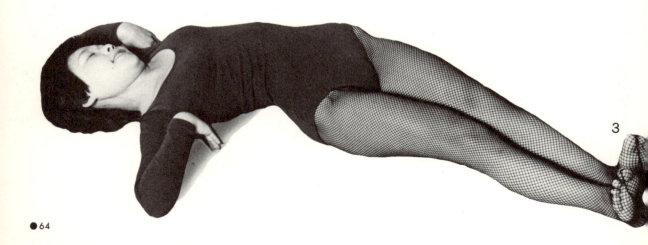

Movements and Breathing Order

1. With both legs together and with fists (thumbs inside) above your head, position your arms to form right angles on either side of your head

2. Inhale, then exhaling, without letting your fists leave the floor, extending your Achilles' tendons, raise both legs straight up till they are at a ninety-degree angle with the floor.

3. Inhaling, then exhaling, lower one leg until it is close to the floor. Inhaling, raise it to a ninety-degree angle again. Repeat, alternating legs, several times (A and B).

4. Return to the position in step 2. Keeping your fists, elbows, and shoulders on the floor, swing both feet to the right until they almost touch the floor. Then, inhaling, raise them both to ninety degrees again. Next, swing them to the left in the same manner (A, B, and C). Return them to the center before lowering them to the floor.

Effects

This exercise strengthens the muscles of the legs and the sides, thus stimulating the liver and stomach and improving circulation in the abdomen.

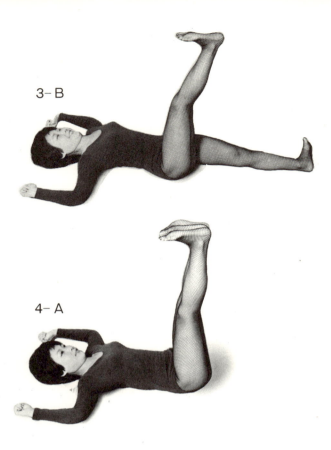

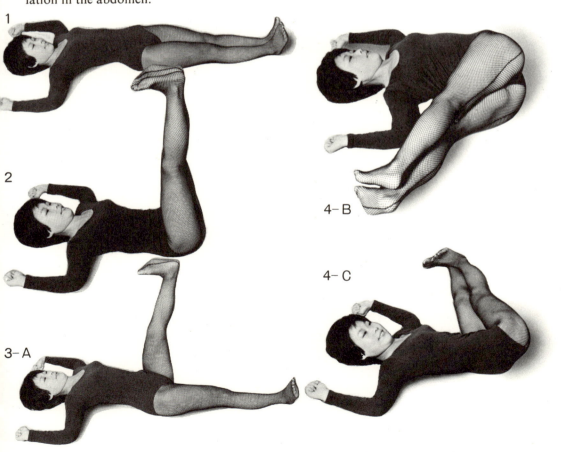

Movements and Breathing Order

1.   Lying on your back, bend both legs backward until your feet lie at the outsides of your buttocks. Stretch both arms on the floor above your head.

2.   Inhale, then exhaling, raise your hips as high as possible without allowing your knees to leave the floor. Then abruptly relax and allow your buttocks to fall to the floor.

Effects

By stimulating and tightening the iliac bone, this exercise eliminates the forward slump caused by weak abdominal muscles and contraction of the muscles of the chest and legs.

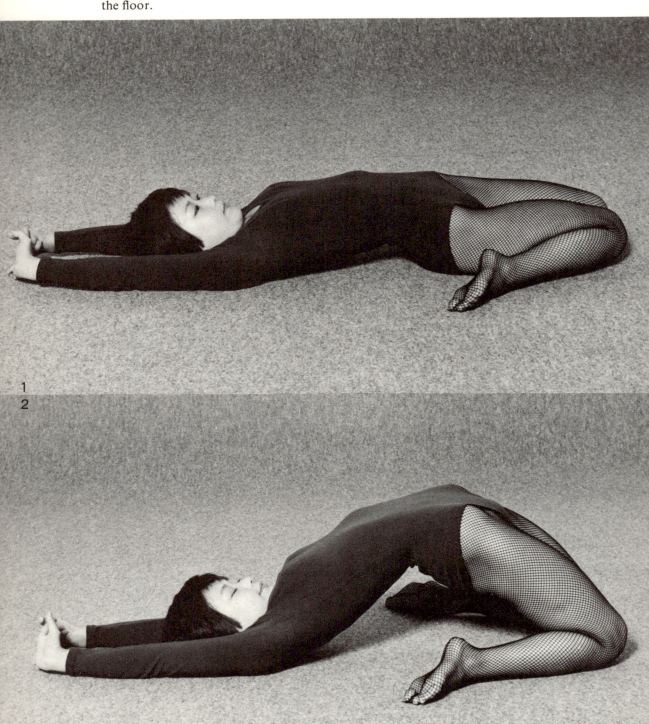

1
2

Movements and Breathing Order

1. Lie on your back with both knees bent and both feet on the floor and spread to about hip width. Bring both hands together at your chest in the prayerful attitude.

2. Inhale and exhale as you raise your body until it is supported only on your head and feet. Breathing deeply, hold this position—with hands till in the prayerful attitude—for a few minutes. Exhaling, slowly lower your body.

Effects

Since it stimulates the muscles of the back and the abdomen, this exercise affects all of the internal organs, strengthens the spinal column, and activates the endocrine system.

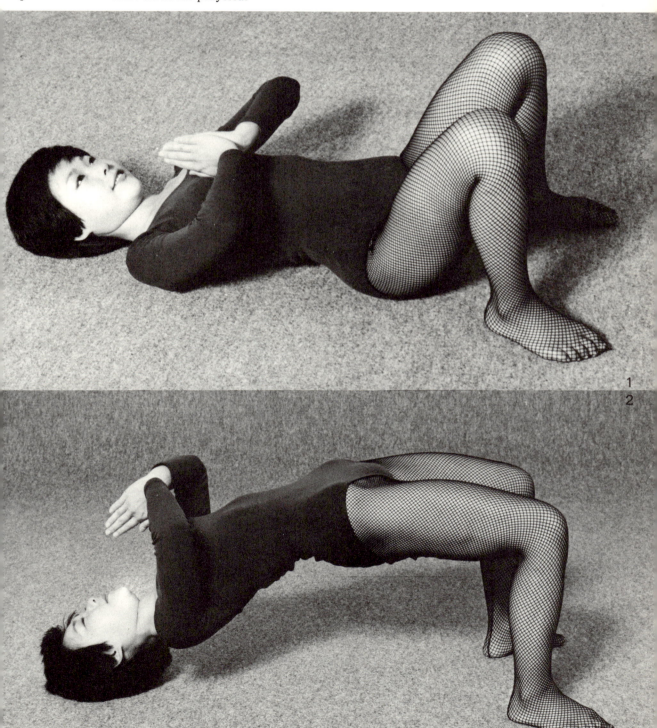

1
2

Movements and Breathing Order

1. Lying on your back, bend both legs back at the knees until your feet lie at the sides of your hips. Grip your ankles in your hands.

2–3. Inhale and exhale and pull both ankles. Tense your entire body and rise without pressing your knees strongly against the floor.

Effects

This exercise improves the elasticity of the abdominal muscles and corrects the old-looking, forward stoop resulting from weakness in those muscles and contraction in the muscles of the thighs.

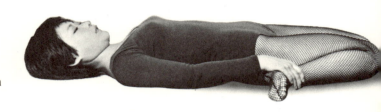

1

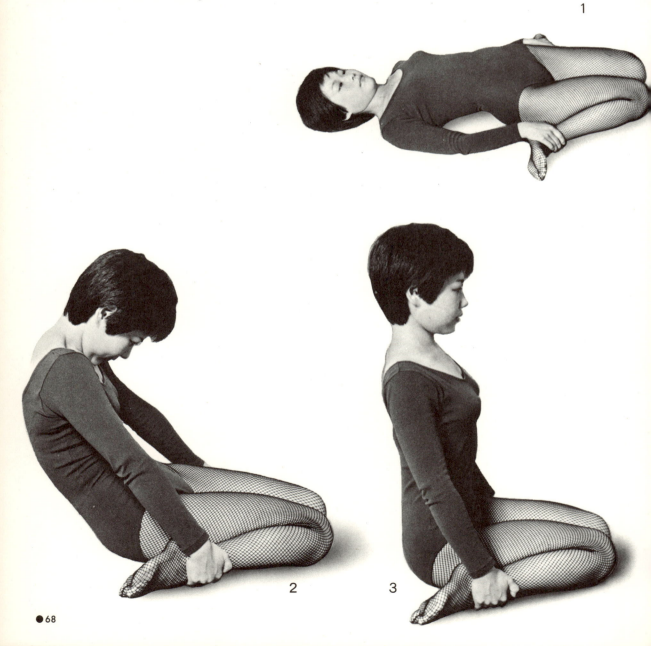

2   3

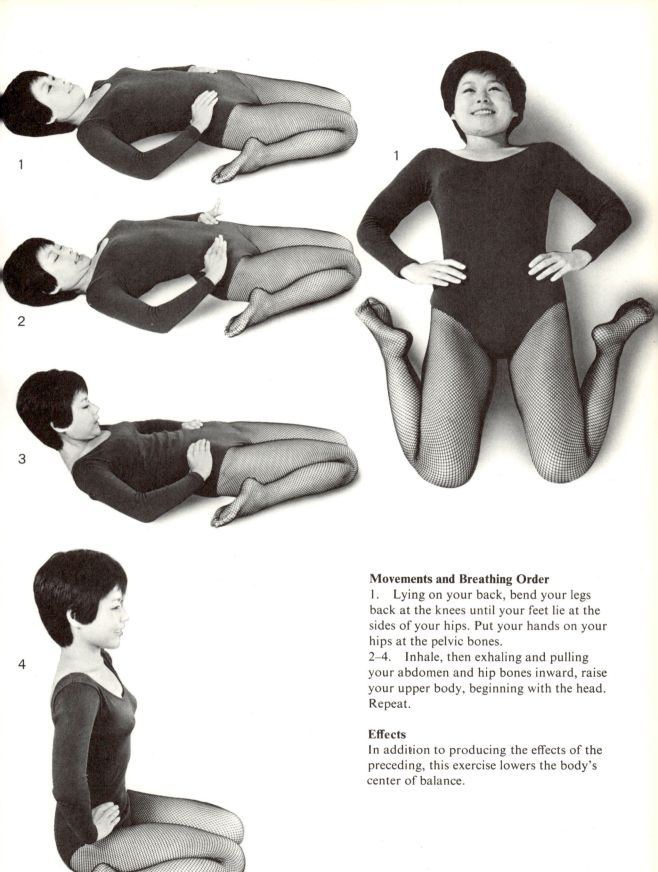

Movements and Breathing Order

1. Lying on your back, bend your legs back at the knees until your feet lie at the sides of your hips. Put your hands on your hips at the pelvic bones.

2–4. Inhale, then exhaling and pulling your abdomen and hip bones inward, raise your upper body, beginning with the head. Repeat.

Effects

In addition to producing the effects of the preceding, this exercise lowers the body's center of balance.

Movements and Breathing Order

1.   Lying on your stomach, extend both arms straight to the sides and bring your legs together. **36**

2.   Inhale and, as you exhale, turning your arms inward (or outward), with both knees and both Achilles' tendons extended, swing your legs to the right, holding them just barely above the floor. At the same time, bend your head until it touches your left shoulder.

3.   Inhaling, return your body to the position in step 1. Then repeat the exercise in the opposite direction.

Effects **37**

This exercise corrects sagging and abnormal placement of internal organs. Swinging your legs to the left and right activates the liver and the stomach.

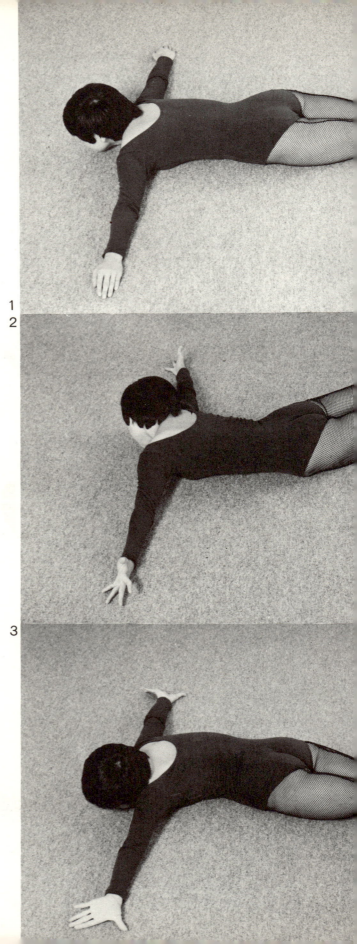

1
2

3

Movements and Breathing Order

1.   Lying on your stomach, put your knees on the floor but raise your hips till your thighs are at a right angle to the floor. Put your chest on the floor and extend both arms straight forward. Inhaling, then exhaling, attempt several times to press your chest still closer against the floor.

2–3.   Putting your hands on the floor beside your chest, raise the upper part of your body and bend backward until you are looking at the ceiling. Inhaling, return to the position in step 1. Exhaling, repeat.

Effects

Since it stretches the abdominal and chest muscles, this exercise eliminates pressure on the internal organs, sagging of the ribs, and contraction and hardening of the chest muscles. It stimulates natural liveliness, self-confidence, and a bright and active personality.

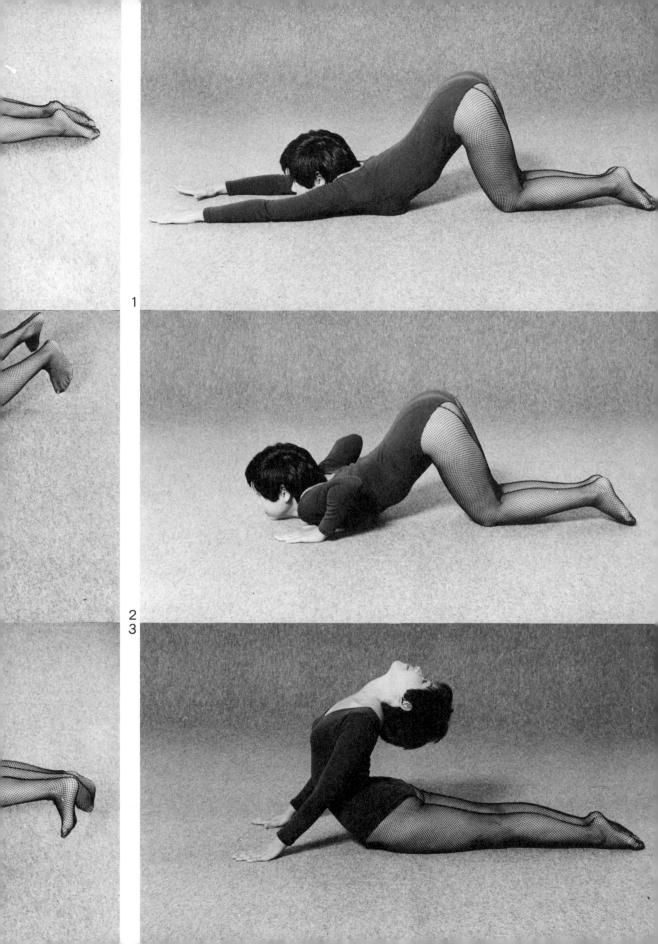

1

2
3

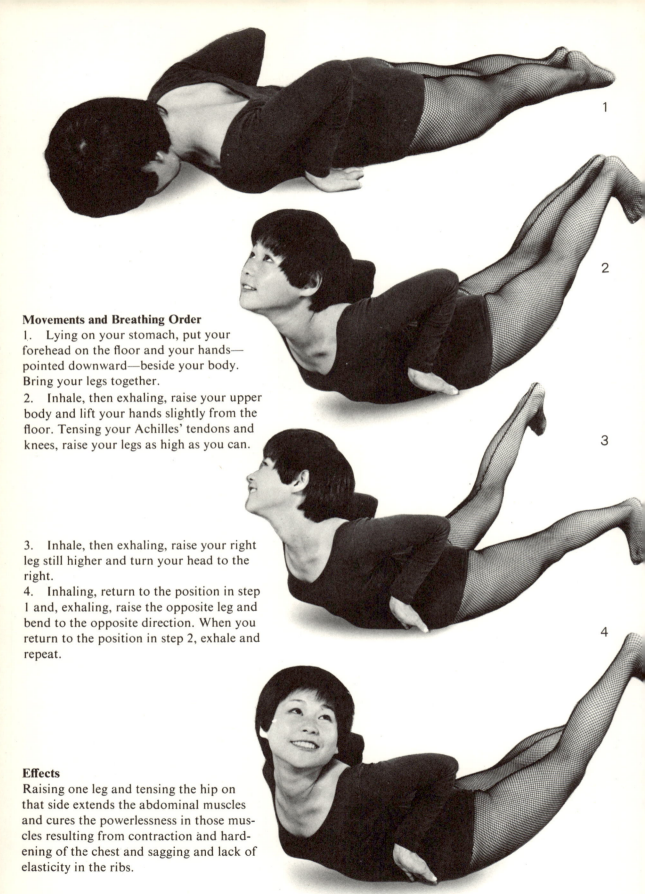

1

2

3

Movements and Breathing Order

1. Lying on your stomach, put your forehead on the floor and your hands—pointed downward—beside your body. Bring your legs together.

2. Inhale, then exhaling, raise your upper body and lift your hands slightly from the floor. Tensing your Achilles' tendons and knees, raise your legs as high as you can.

3. Inhale, then exhaling, raise your right leg still higher and turn your head to the right.

4. Inhaling, return to the position in step 1 and, exhaling, raise the opposite leg and bend to the opposite direction. When you return to the position in step 2, exhale and repeat.

4

Effects

Raising one leg and tensing the hip on that side extends the abdominal muscles and cures the powerlessness in those muscles resulting from contraction and hardening of the chest and sagging and lack of elasticity in the ribs.

Nearsightedness, Astigmatism, and Other Disorders in Vision

Goals and Effects

Myopia—or nearsightedness—is of two kinds: axial (caused by congestion and hyperacidity of the blood) and refractory (caused by stiffness of the ciliary muscles). Obviously because of its complicated causes, such a condition cannot be, cured by treating the eyes alone.

The following kinds of exercises may be used to treat various eye conditions. Correcting twists in the neck, sagging scalp, and lowering of the shoulder blades has a salutary effect on crossed eyes. Treating shoulder blades that are too high or abnormal strength and weakness in the arms cures astigmatism. Hypermetropia is cured in the same way as myopia. Poor sight caused by aging requires the kind of exercises employed in general rejuvenation of the body.

In all of these exercises, total relaxation of the arms, shoulders, and neck is especially important, as tension in these parts of the body causes blood congestion in the eyes and brings about fatigue.

Movements and Breathing Order

Inhaling and then exhaling, roll your eyeballs up, down, right, left, diagonally up right, diagonally right down, diagonally left up, and diagonally left down. If it is possible, hold each position a few seconds then suddenly return to the original eye position (A–H). Then, inhaling and exhaling, roll your eyes as far as possible to the right and left. It is important to roll your eyes and farther in all directions than you do in ordinary vision, since this stimulates the muscles, relieves fatigue, and increases the eyes' limitations of motion.

Effects

Rolling the eyes in this way relieves rigidity and irregularity in the muscles related to the eyes.

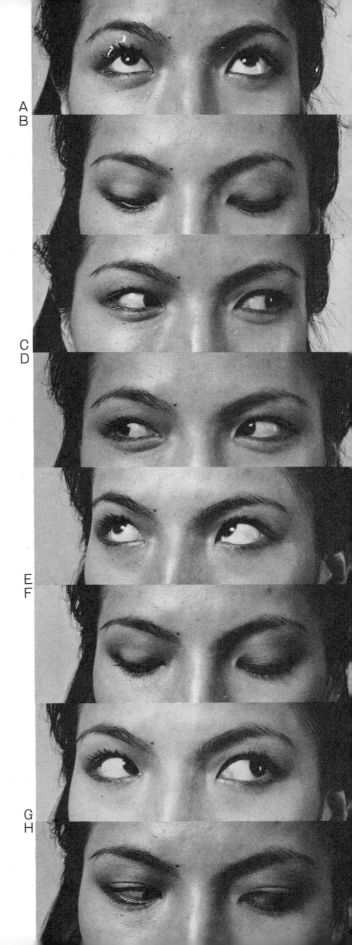

A
B
C
D
E
F
G
H

Movements and Breathing Order

1. Focusing on nothing, relax your face and direct your vision into space.
2. Exhaling, turn both eyes to the tip of your nose. Hold them in this position for a few seconds then suddenly relax. Repeat two or three times.

Effects

This exercise corrects imbalance between the sets of muscles for the eyes and improves the eyes' self-control capability. It lubricates the eyes by stimulating the tear glands and ducts. Further, by equalizing stress in the eyes, face, and mind, it causes facial relaxation and makes you subconsciously aware of mental tensions.

Movements and Breathing Order ▶

1. After warming your palms by rubbing them together, cup them over your eyes. Feel the warmth penetrating deep into your eyes and relaxing your ciliary muscles. To achieve these ends, you must relax the muscles of your shoulders, neck, and face and smile.
2. Inhale then exhale with force. Wink as hard as you can with one eye, then with the other. Repeat several times (A and B).

Effects

These exercises stimulate circulation. Winking stimulates the tear glands and relaxes the eyes.

1 2

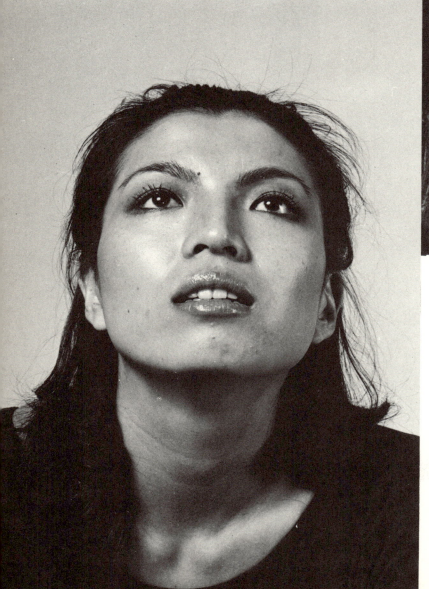
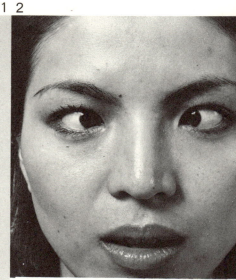

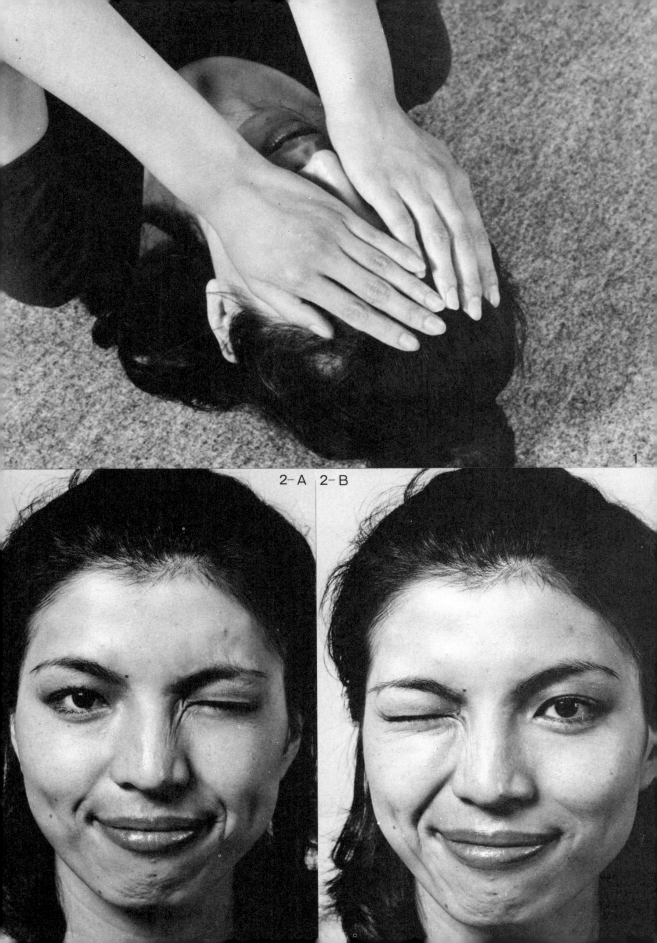

2-A 2-B

1

Movements and Breathing Order

1. Press the area around the eyes and the interior of the orbits (A, B, C, and D).
2. Using the thumbs and forefingers, exert a squeezing pressure on the area from the forehead to the tip of the nose (A and B).

Effects

By stimulating the area around the eyes, these exercises improve circulation, relieve eye fatigue, and prevent myopia.

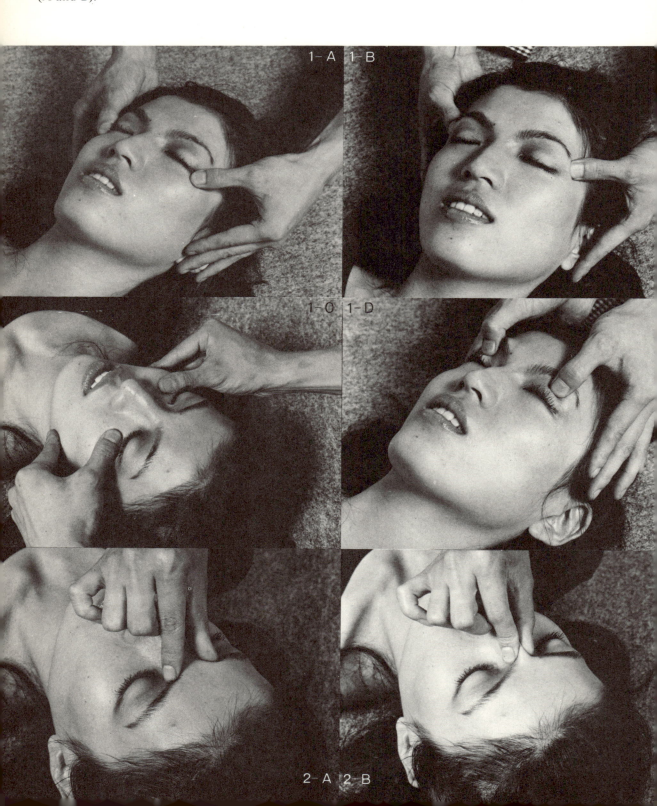

Movements and Breathing Order (Six Points or *tsubo*)

1. With the fingers locked behind the head, press with your thumbs on the spot just below the ear lobes. Pressure must be directed toward the eyes. Then stimulate with a squeezing motion (point one; 1A and 1B).
2. Press and squeeze the point at the middle of the muscle running from the area below the ear diagonally forward and downward (point two).
3. Press upward and rub with your index fingers on the points under the chin (point three, 3).
4. Press and rub in an upward direction along the cheeks from beside the nose outward (point four, 4A and 4B).
5. With fingers locked behind the head, press and rub the temples in the direction of the eyes with your thumbs (point five).
6. Press and rub on the hollow on the back of the head just at ear height and immediately behind the eyes.

Effects

Although many *tsubo* all over the body are related to the eyes, these six are the closest to the eyes. Treatment on them improves circulation and stimulates the tear glands.

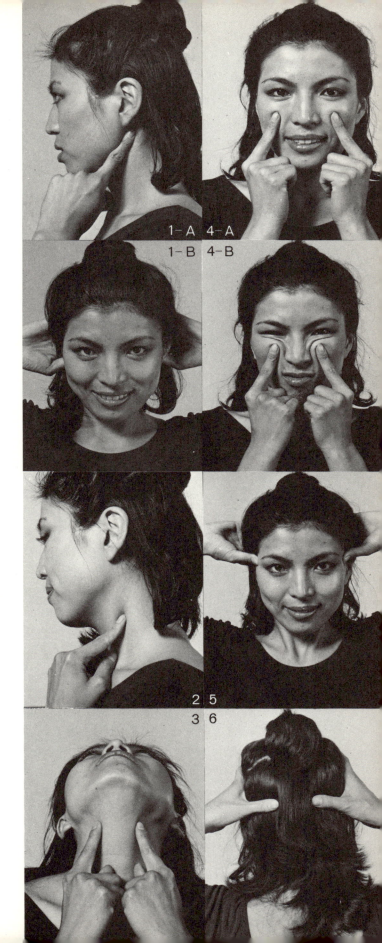

1-A 4-A
1-B 4-B
2 5
3 6

Movements and Breathing Order

1.   Lying on your back, outstretch your right arm (fist clenched with thumbs inside) straight to the side.

2–3.   Inhale and, as you exhale, rolling the fist inward and outward, outstretch your arm, then relax. Repeat as you gradually raise the right arm over your head. Repeat with the other arm.

Effects

Twisting the wrist stimulates muscles related to the eyes and relaxes the arms, shoulders, and neck.

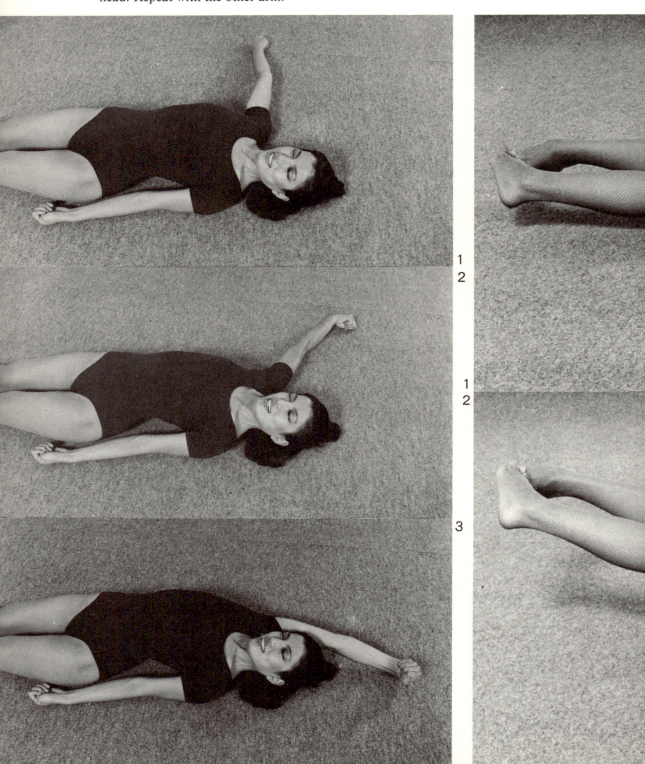

Movements and Breathing Order

1. Lying on your back, stretch both arms (fists clenched) over your head. Your legs are straight, and your feet are turned inward.

2. Raise your feet about thirty centimeters off the floor. Turning your wrists inward and outward, raise and lower your legs and roll your eyes upward. Inhale when you raise them and exhale and roll your eyes downward when you lower them.

Effects

Raising and lowering your legs with your feet turned inward in this fashion increase abdominal pressure. Turning your wrists inward and outward stimulates the tear glands and the shoulder blades.

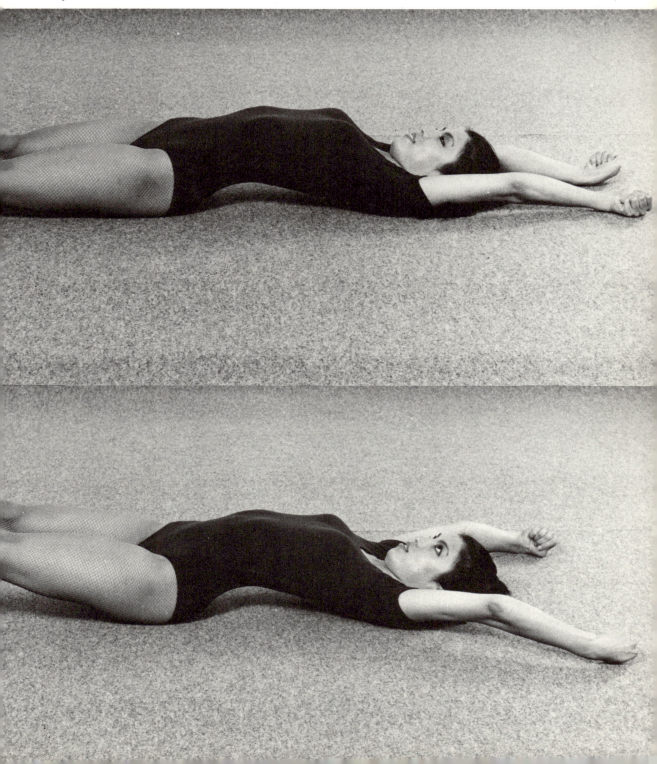

Movements and Breathing Order

1. Sit straight up with arms and legs outstretched parallel and straight forward and with your Achilles' tendons extended. Clench your fists.

2. Inhale. As you exhale, lean backward and raise your legs from the floor to put your body in a V shape tilted about forty-five degrees from the floor.

3. Inhale. As you exhale, twisting your hands inward and outward, gradually open your arms to the side.

Effects

Putting your body in this V shape develops abdominal pressure. Opening your arms while rotating your wrists adjusts your shoulder blades.

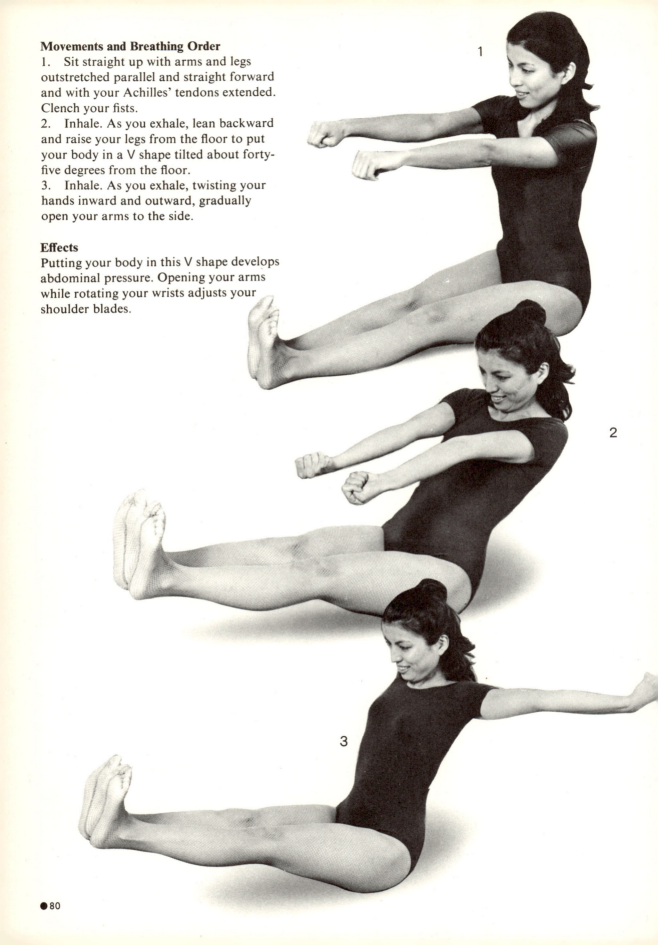

Movements and Breathing Order

1. Kneeling in the *seiza* position, with feet spread, lower your buttocks to the floor and then bend over backward until your upper body lies on the floor (this position is called *wariza*).

2. With the fingers of both hands interlocked and your palms turned outward, outstretch your arms.

3. Inhaling, then exhaling, raise your shoulders and hips until your body is supported by your head and lower legs only.

4–5. Inhale. Then, as you exhale, lower both arms to the floor over your head. Raise them again as you inhale. When you bring your arms upward, roll your eyes upward; and downward when you lower your arms.

6–7. Inhale then exhale as you swing your arms to the right. Exhale as you bring them back to the center. Then inhale and exhale as you swing them to the left. Repeat. Your eyes should roll left with the leftward and right with the rightward swing.

Effects

This exercise relieves contractions of the superficial muscles of the chest and legs, strengthens the hips, and limbers the shoulders and neck. The forward bend has a good effect on visual weakness.

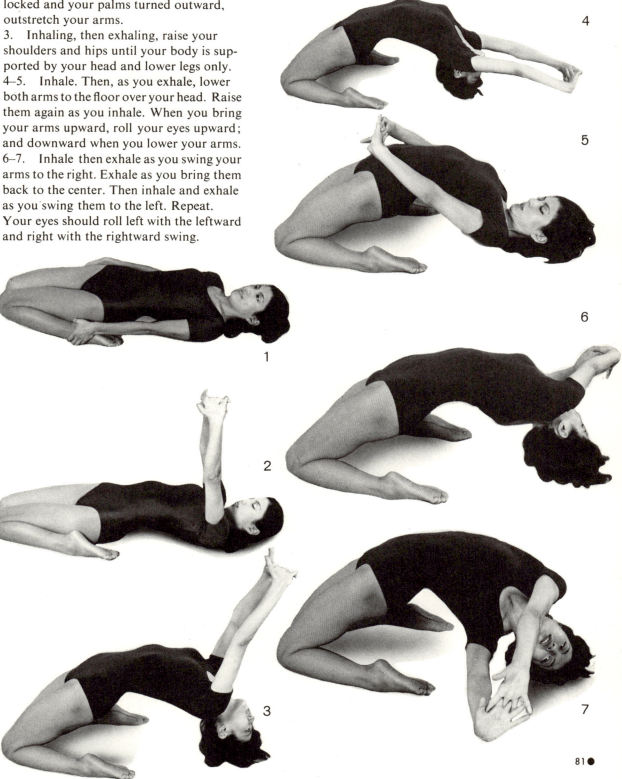

Movements and Breathing Order

1. Lying on your back with legs bent and knees raised, clench your fists and put your arms on the floor with forearms raised above your head at right angles.

2. Inhale and, as you exhale, raise your hips off the floor.

3–4. Inhale and, as you exhale, turn your fists inward and roll your head to the right. Then, twisting your wrists outward, turn your face to the left. Repeat.

Effects

Twisting the wrists stimulates the eyes. Raising your hips and turning your neck right and left limbers your shoulders and neck, strengthens your hips, and relaxes your eyes.

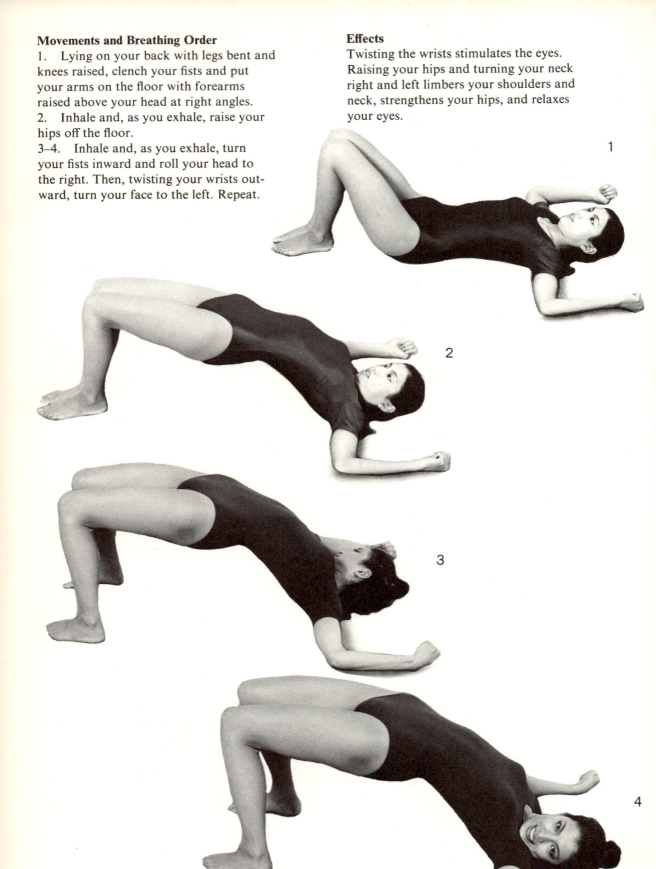

Movements and Breathing Order

1.　Lying on your back with legs bent and knees raised, press the six eye points with both hands (the model is pressing the first point).

2.　Inhale and, as you exhale, raise your upper body (3).

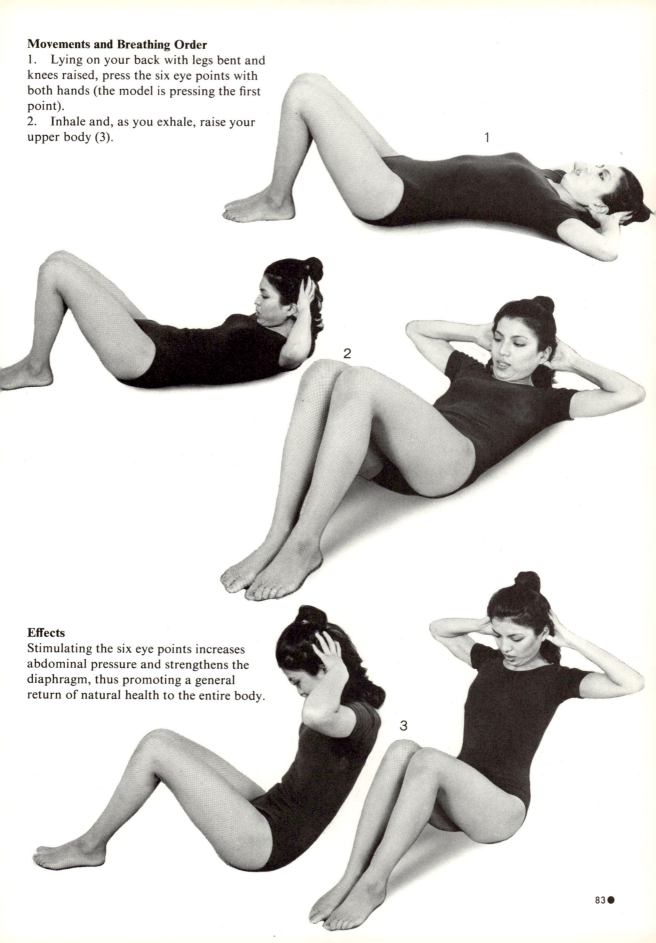

Effects

Stimulating the six eye points increases abdominal pressure and strengthens the diaphragm, thus promoting a general return of natural health to the entire body.

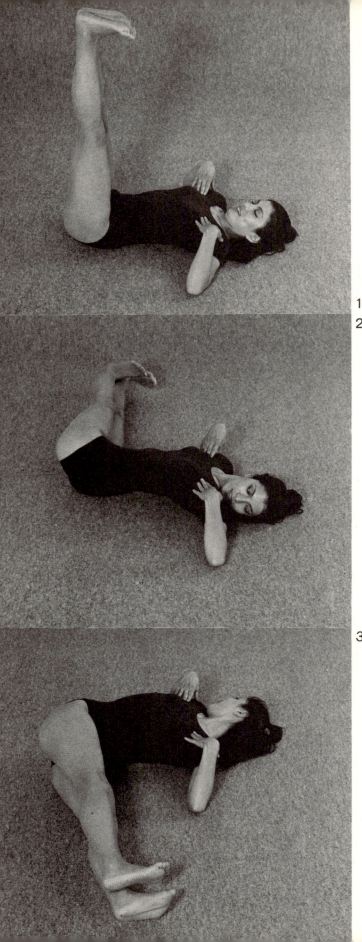

Movements and Breathing Order

1. Lying on your back, put your hands on your chest and raise both legs together to an angle of ninety degrees with the floor. Extend your Achilles' tendons.

2. Inhale and, as you exhale, turn your head to the left and lower both legs to the right. Your left shoulder must not leave the floor.

3. As you inhale, return to the position in step 1. Then, exhaling, lower your legs to the left as you turn your head to the right. Your eyes must turn in the same direction as your head.

Effects

Twists to the right and left limber the shoulders, neck, and hips. This will cure slight abnormalities caused by constipation.

Movements and Breathing Order ▶

1. Lying on your back, put your arms diagonally to your sides. Inhale and, as you exhale, raise your legs and lower your feet to the floor above your head.

2–3. Inhale and, as you exhale, turn your hips to the left and your head to the right. inhaling, return to the position in step 1. Then, as you exhale, turn your hips to the right and your head to the left. Repeat and return slowly to the supine position.

Effects

This plow pose relieves blood congestion in the lower abdomen and limbers the spinal column. Lowering your buttocks to the right and left relieves contraction in the sides of the abdomen and eliminates blood congestion in the neck and shoulders.

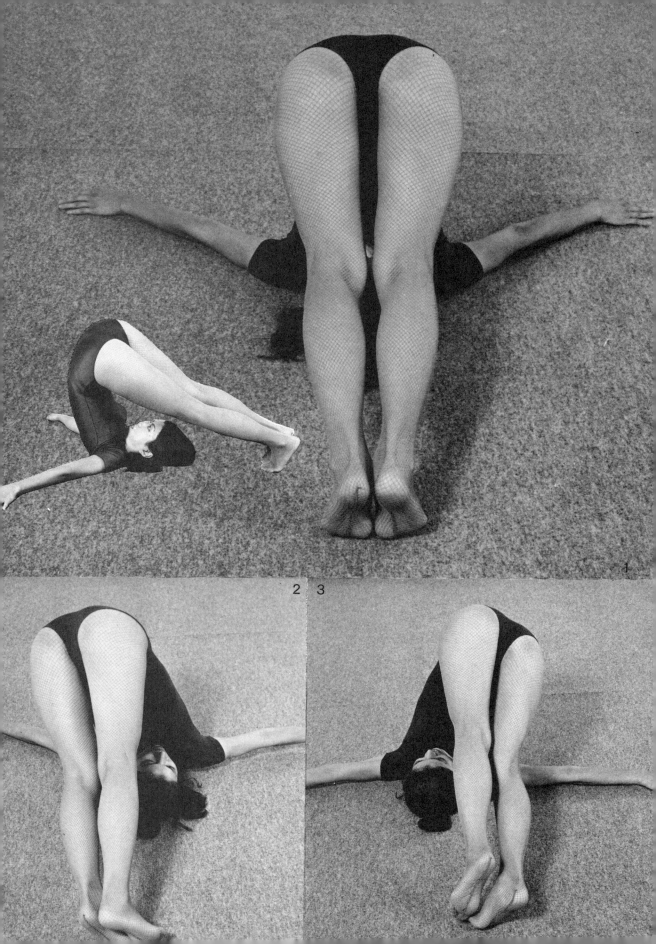

1

2 3

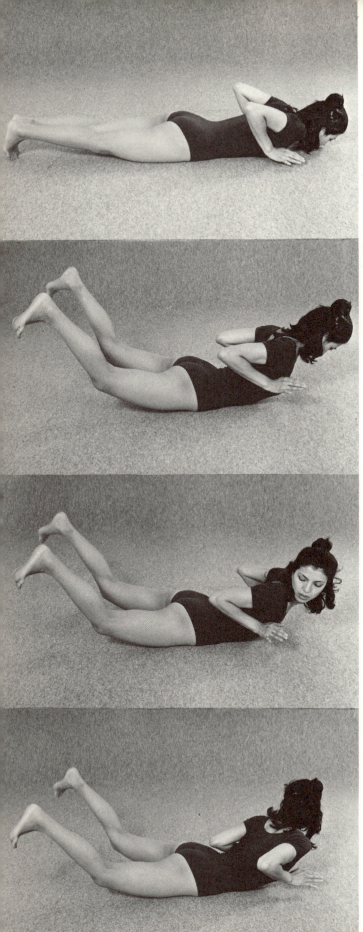

Movements and Breathing Order

1. Lying on your stomach with your hands under your shoulders, bend your elbows as if you were trying to bring your shoulder blades together.

2. Inhale and, as you exhale, raise both legs. Lift your hands from the floor.

3–4. Exhaling, turn your upper body to the right. Inhaling, return to the position in step 2. Then, exhaling again, turn your upper body to the left.

Effects

This has the same strengthening effect on the kidneys as the cobra pose. Further, it regulates the shoulder blades.

Movements and Breathing Order ▶

1. Lying on your stomach, lock the fingers of both hands behind your back and turn your palms outward.

2. Having your partner hold your feet, inhale. Then, as you exhale, raise your upper body and bend your neck backward.

3–4. Inhale and, as you exhale, turn your upper body to the right. As you inhale, return to the position in step 1. Then, as you exhale, turn your upper body to the left. Your eyes must turn to the right when your head turns right and to the left when it turns left.

Effects

The effects, the same as those of the preceding exercise, are intensified because of the assistance of a partner.

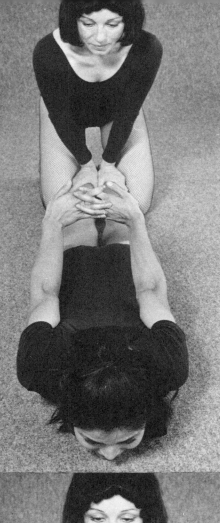

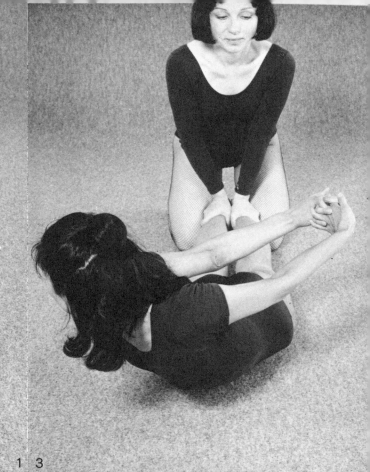

1 3

2 4

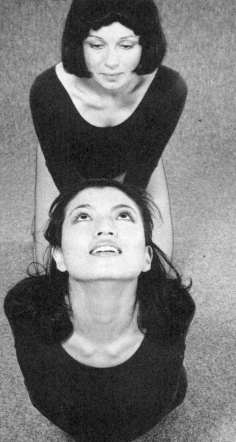

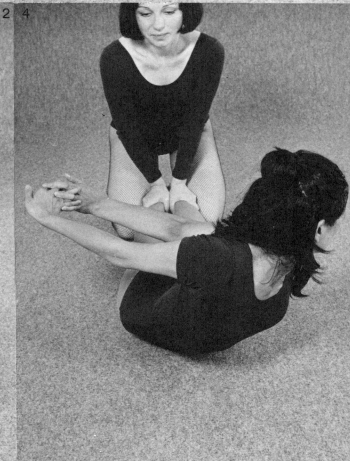

Movements and Breathing Order

1. Kneel with your hands joined under your chin, your knees at right angles to the floor, and your buttocks raised high.

2. As you inhale then exhale, raise and outstretch your left leg.

3–4. Inhale and, as you exhale, lower your left leg and your buttocks to the right. As you inhale, return to the position in step 2. Repeat the exercise with the right leg. Bring your leg as close to the floor as possible each time and do not allow your elbows to leave the floor. Turn your eyes in the direction of the lowered leg.

Effects

This variation of the cat pose limbers the spinal column and corrects forward stoop. By stimulating the kidneys, it adjusts the shoulder blades.

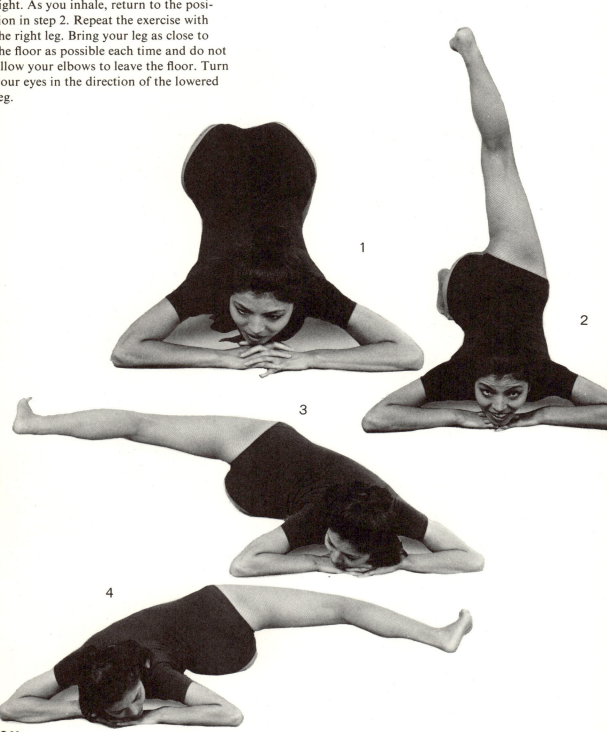

Movements and Breathing Order

1. Lying on our stomach, put your elbows on the floor. Then, as you inhale and exhale, raise your hips so that your body is supported by only your elbows and toes.

2–3. Inhale and, as you exhale, move your body forward. Then, as you inhale again, move your body rearward. Repeat. Your eye movement must be synchronized with the movement of your body.

Effects

Supporting your body on the elbows and toes relieves congestion in the abdomen and limbers the shoulder blades. It is especially important in increasing your ability to move your body up and down and in strengthening the abdomen.

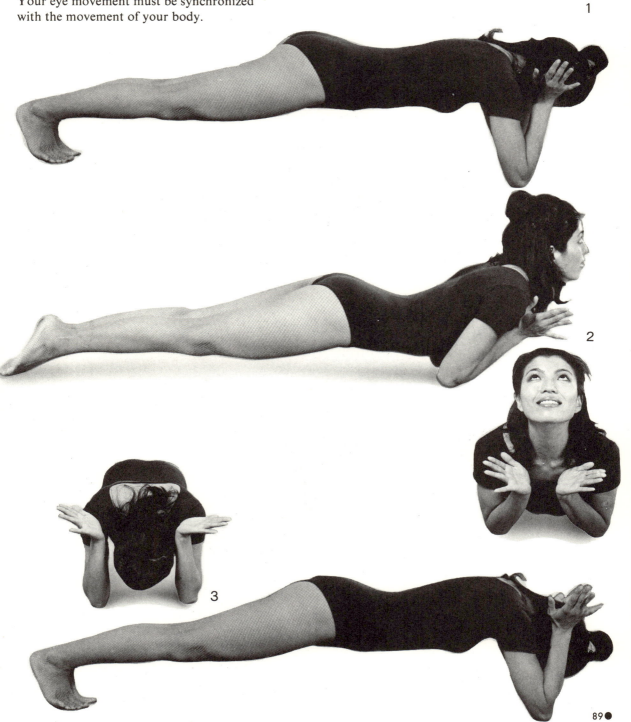

89

Movements and Breathing Order

1. Lying face down, put your hands—fingers pointed outward—on the floor to your sides. Your upper arms should be straight and fully extended. Put only the toes of your feet on the floor. Inhale and, as you exhale, raise your body so that it is supported only on your toes and hands.

2. Inhale and, as you exhale, slide your body to the right as if you were pressing your right shoulder blade with your left one. Inhaling, return your body to the position in step 1.

3. Repeat, moving your body to the left. Orient your eyes in the direction in which your body moves.

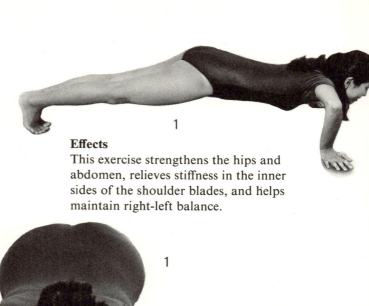

1

Effects

This exercise strengthens the hips and abdomen, relieves stiffness in the inner sides of the shoulder blades, and helps maintain right-left balance.

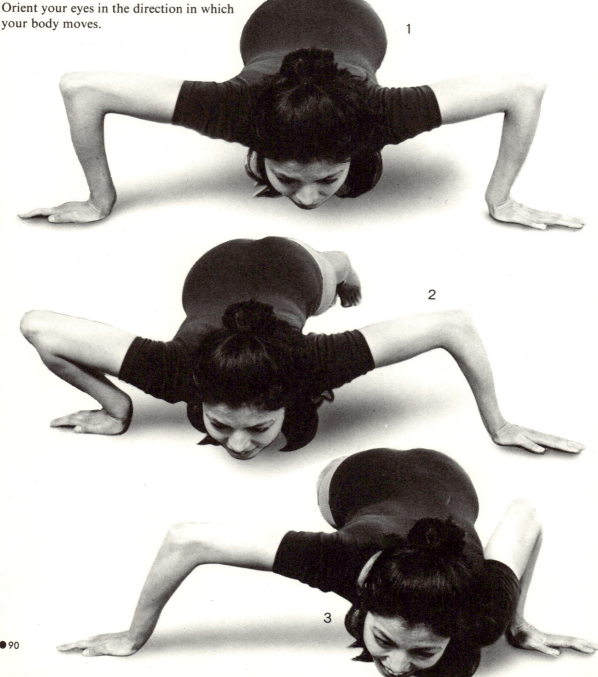

1

2

3

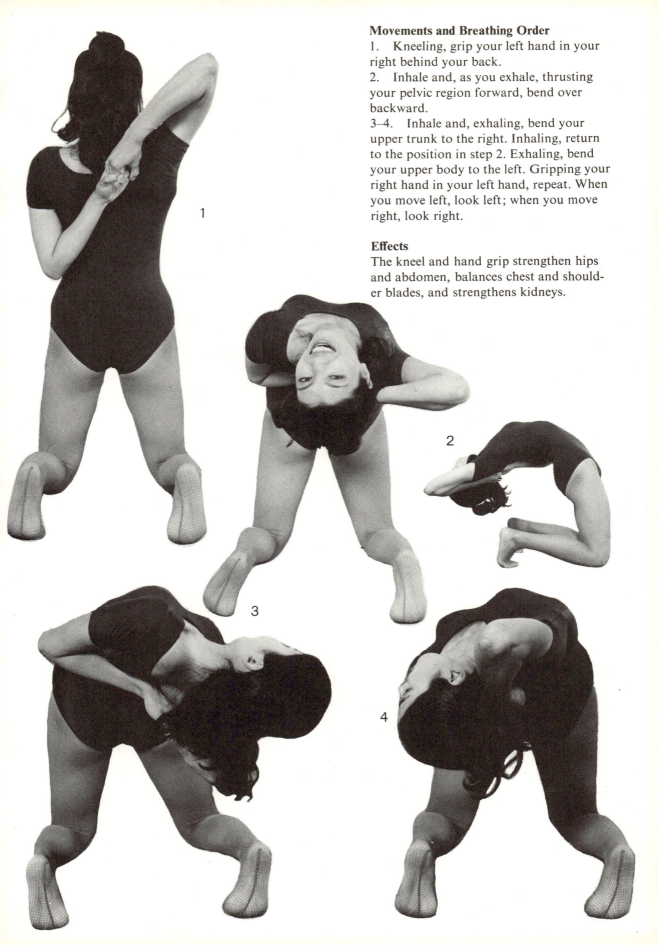

Movements and Breathing Order

1. Kneeling, grip your left hand in your right behind your back.
2. Inhale and, as you exhale, thrusting your pelvic region forward, bend over backward.
3–4. Inhale and, exhaling, bend your upper trunk to the right. Inhaling, return to the position in step 2. Exhaling, bend your upper body to the left. Gripping your right hand in your left hand, repeat. When you move left, look left; when you move right, look right.

Effects

The kneel and hand grip strengthen hips and abdomen, balances chest and shoulder blades, and strengthens kidneys.

1

2

3

4

Movements and Breathing Order

1. Kneeling, press on the six eye points with the fingers of both hands (the model is pressing the first point).
2. Inhale and, as you exhale, lean backward, thrusting your pelvic region forward.
3–4. Inhale and, as you exhale, bend your upper body to the right. Inhaling, return to the position in step 2. Then in-hale and, as you exhale, turn your upper body to the left. Repeat.

Effects

While stimulating the kidneys, this exercise stimulates the vital points (*tsubo*) for the eyes as well.

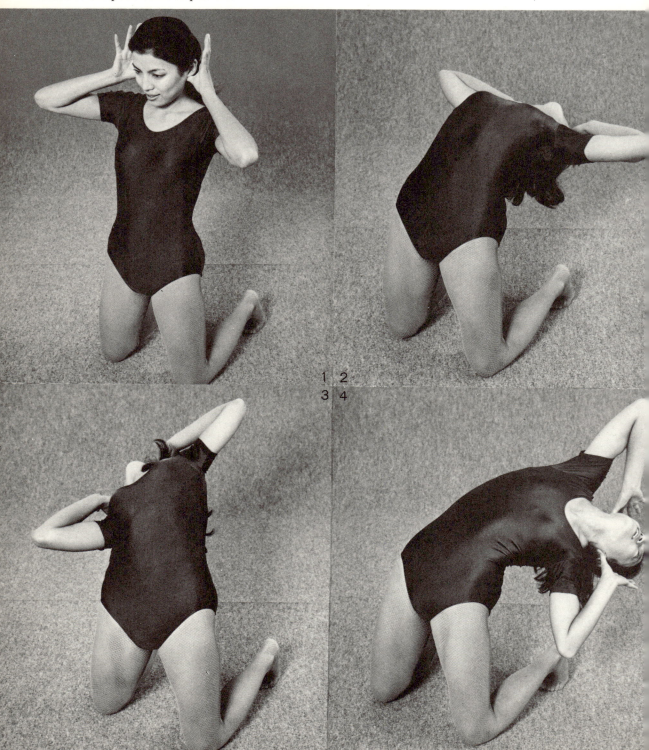

1 2
3 4

Abnormalities in the Ears and Nose

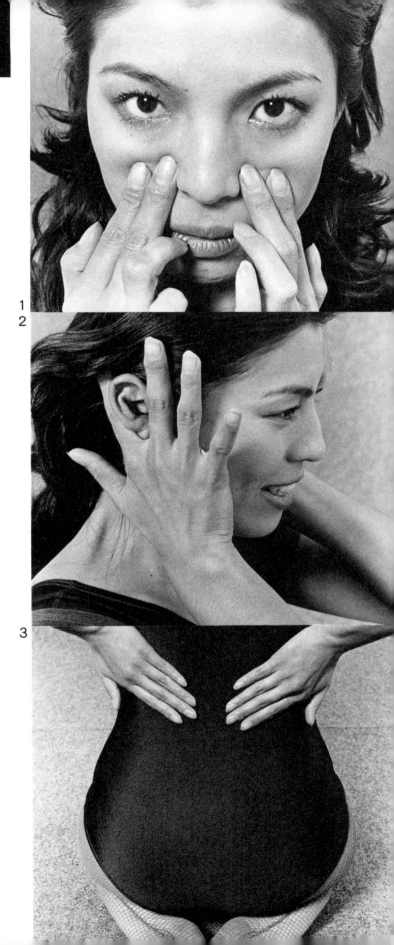

Goals and Effects

Yoga exercises to correct troubles in the ears and nose concentrate on movements to lower the pubic bone and to twist the neck. For people with bad ears, bending of the neck and exercises to strengthen the lateral abdominal muscles, as well as movements to stretch the shorter leg are recommended. People with nose trouble should avoid overeating.

Ear trouble may be divided into two major categories: irregularities between the outer and middle ears and those between the middle and inner ears. In young people, ringing of the ears and poor hearing are caused by bad posture, sickness, or drug abuse. In old people, nervous fatigue, contraction, and stiffness around the ears are the major causes of poor hearing. Many people with poor hearing suffer from abnormalities in the intestines or the kidneys; consequently, the exercises take the internal organs into consideration, though some of them concentrate on stretching the muscles of the undersides of the feet and of the neck.

Movements and Breathing Order

1. Rub upward on both sides of the nostrils with the index and middle fingers.

Effects

This improves circulation and relieves blood congestion.

Movements and Breathing Order

2. Rub and stroke your ears, which are held between the index and middle fingers of each hand.

Effects

This relieves stiffness and contraction around the ears, eases blood congestion, and improves circulation to the kidneys.

Movements and Breathing Order

3. Rub and stimulate with both hands the area of the back where the kidneys are located.

Effects

Stimulating the kidneys improves the functioning of the ears.

Movements and Breathing Order

1. Sitting on the floor with your legs outstretched in front of you, put both hands on the floor behind you and lean backward. Bend first one knee then the other and put the foot of the bent leg on the knee of the outstretched one.

2. Inhale and, as you exhale, roll over to the right, turning your head to the left and then roll to the left, turning your head to the right.

Effects

Rolling to the side in this way stimulates the lateral abdominal muscles and the sacral vertebrae while improving the functioning of the kidneys, ears, and nose.

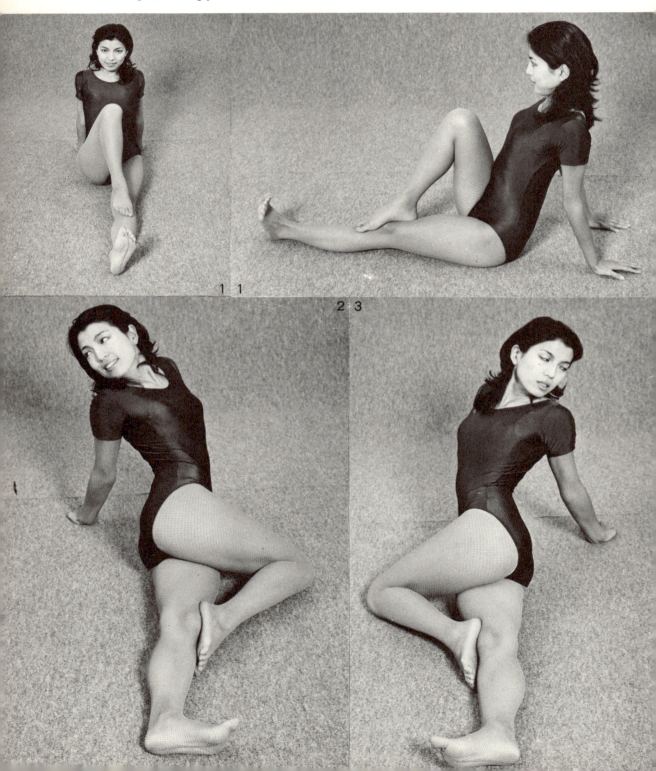

Movements and Breathing Order

1. Lying on your back, stretch your arms—fists clenched, thumbs inside—over your head.

2–3. Bend your knees. Inhale and, as you exhale, raise your hips from the floor.

4. When you have fully exhaled, thrusting your hips upward, kick both feet forward and allow your buttocks to fall on the floor. Inhale.

Effects

Clenching the fists and outstretching the arms relieve tension in the shoulders and neck. Dropping the buttocks to the floor relieves congestion in the pubic bone, corrects faulty positioning, and improves the functioning of the nose.

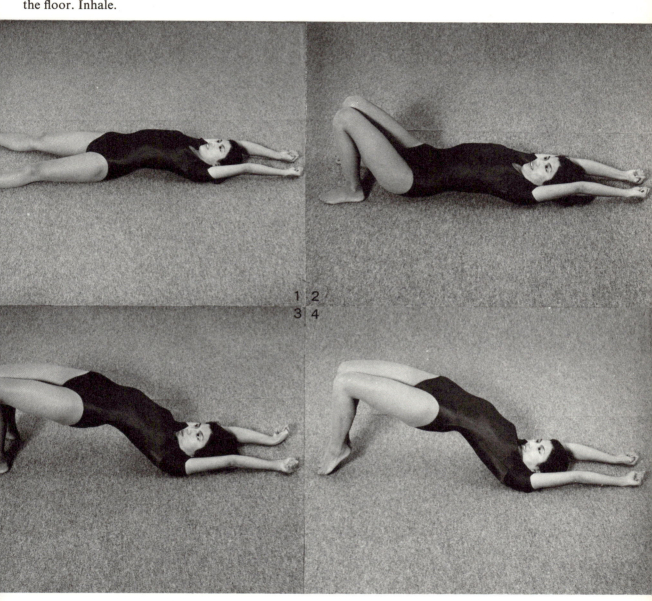

Movements and Breathing Order

1.   Lying on your back, put your elbows on the floor, point your toes upward, and extend your Achilles' tendons. Inhale and, as you exhale, raise your chest and lift your feet slightly from the floor.

2.   Inhale and, as you exhale, turn your head and feet to the right.

3.   As you inhale, return your head and feet to the middle position. As you exhale turn your head and feet to the left. Repeat.

Effects

Raising your chest corrects the positioning of your shoulder blades and relieves congestion. Turning your feet to the right and left stimulates circulation in the neck and improves the functioning of the ears and nose.

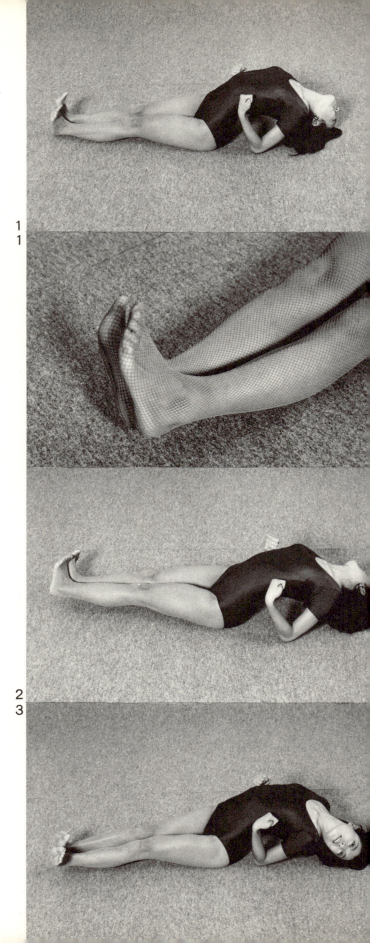

1
1

2
3

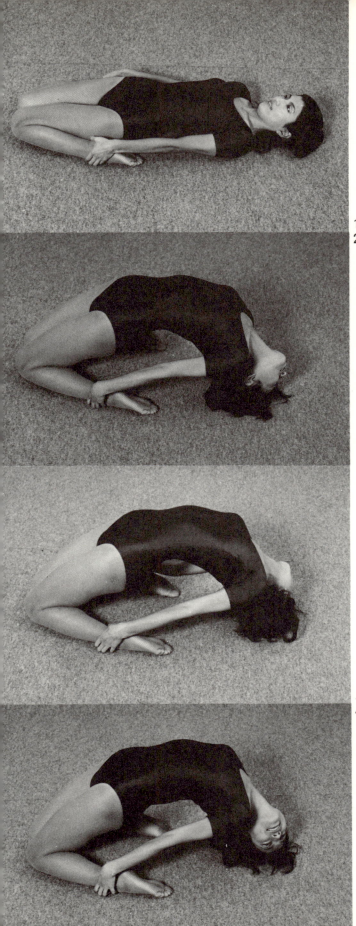

Movements and Breathing Order

1. Kneel in the *seiza* position with your feet outside your buttocks. Lower your buttocks to the floor between your feet and grip both ankles. Lower your upper body to the floor.

2. Inhale and, as you exhale, raise your chest and hips so that your head and lower legs support your body.

3. Inhale and, as you exhale, turn your head to the right.

4. Inhale and return to the middle position. Then, as you exhale, turn your head to the left. Repeat.

Effects

Raising your shoulder and hips increases abdominal pressure, and the turns to the left and the right relieve blood congestion in the sides of the neck and prevent stiffening in the area of the ears.

1
2

3
4

Movements and Breathing Order

1. Lying on your back with your knees bent, put your hands on the floor under your shoulders with fingers pointed toward your feet.
2. Inhale and, as you exhale, raise your hips, chest, and head.
3. Inhale, and as you exhale, roll your hips to the right.
4. Inhale and return to the middle position. Then, as you exhale, roll your hips to the left.

Effects

Raising your hips, chest, and head relieves stiffness in the lateral abdomen and the chest and especially in the muscles of the neck. In addition, it improves circulation to the ears and nose.

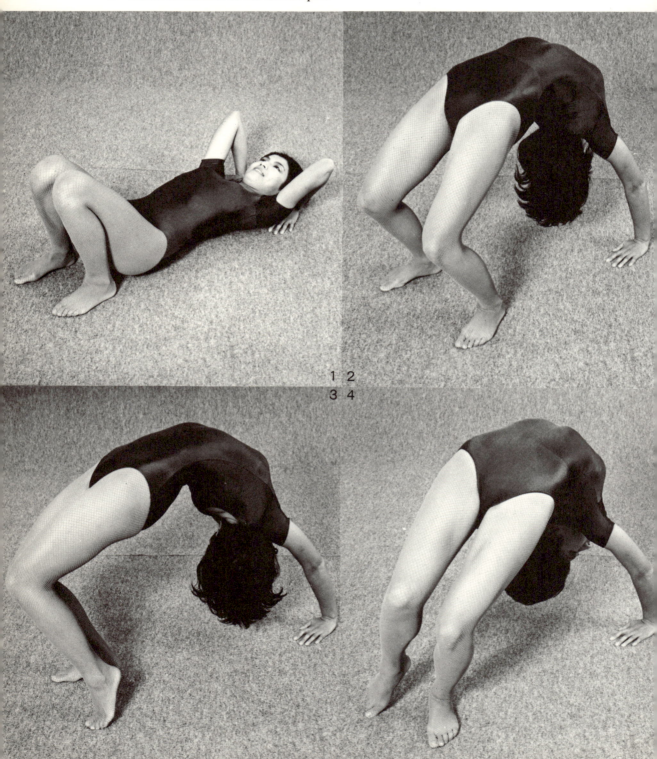

Movements and Breathing Order

1. With feet spread and without bending your knees, bend forward and put your hands on the floor slightly forward of your shoulders.

2. As you inhale, raise your buttocks high and lower your head between your arms.

3. Exhaling forcefully, lower your body so that your pelvic region slides across the floor and your head and trunk rise upward and backward.

Effects

Extending and contracting the muscles in the hips and abdomen improve the functions of the interior organs and lower the body's center of weight. Stretching the neck outward and upward relieves tension in and around the neck.

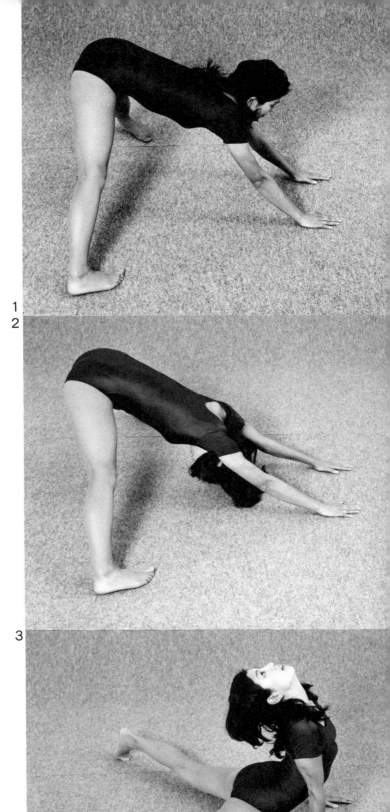

1

2

3

Movements and Breathing Order

1. Crouch with knees and hands on the floor.
2. Inhale and, as you exhale, bend your elbows and lower your chest so that it slides across the floor.
3. Inhale and, as you exhale, raise your right leg.
4. Inhaling, return to the position in step 2. Then, exhaling, raise your left leg.

Effects

Sliding your chest across the floor corrects the placement of the shoulder blades. Raising the legs improves the functioning of the kidneys and stimulates the ears.

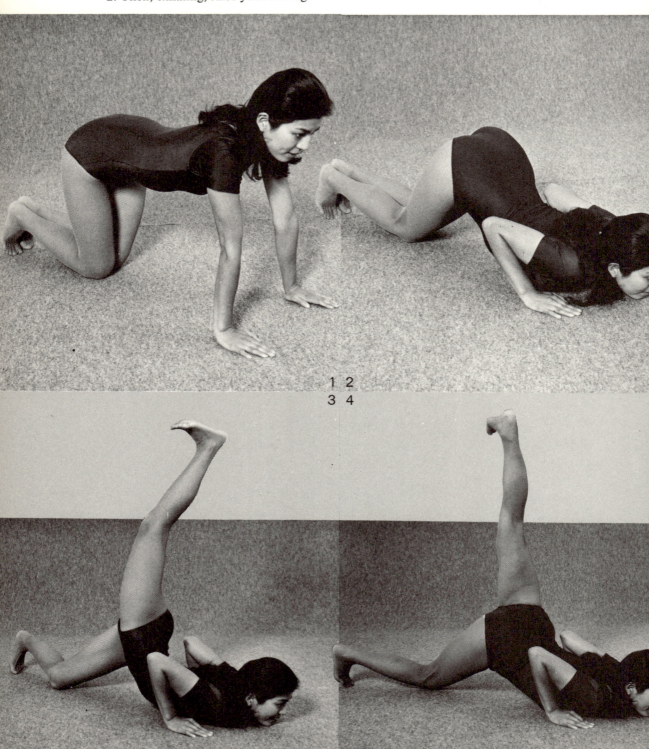

1 2
3 4

Movements and Breathing Order

1.   Kneel in the cat pose with one arm outstretched in front of you and the other bent so that your hand rests under your chin.

2.   Inhale and, exhaling, outstretch one of your legs.

3.   Inhale and, as you exhale, roll over and bring the outstretched leg far to one side. Repeat with the other side.

Effects

Extending one arm and one leg relieves contraction in the area below the shoulder blades and congestion in the hips. In addition, it improves the functioning of the nose and ears.

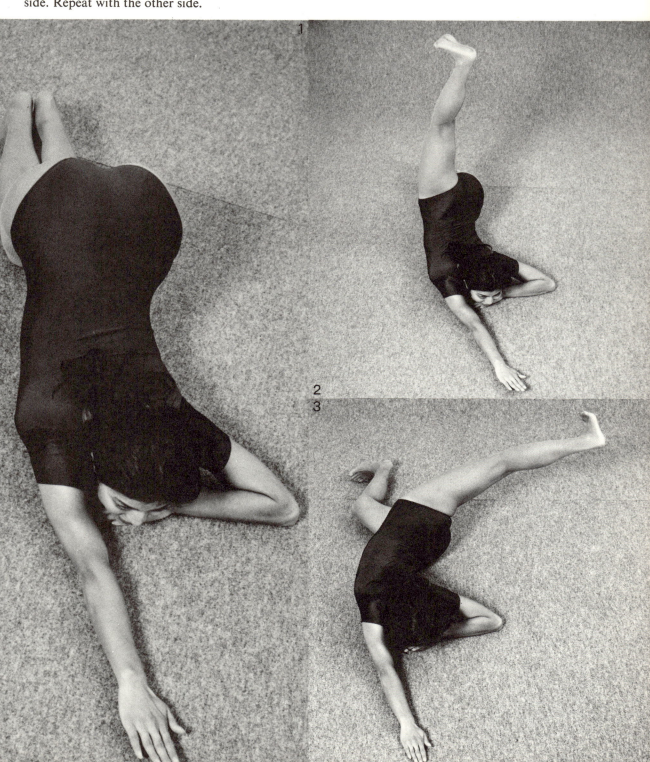

Movements and Breathing Order

1. Lying on your stomach grip both ankles from the inner side. Inhale and, as you exhale, raise your upper body by pulling your ankles.

2–3. Inhale and, as you exhale, turn your face to the right. Inhale and return your head to the central position. Then, exhaling, turn your head to the left (2-A and B, 3-A and B).

Effects

By fully expanding it, this exercise relieves congestion in the abdomen. In addition, it corrects forward stoop and has an effect on all of the internal organs. Turning your face from side to side relieves stiffness of the neck.

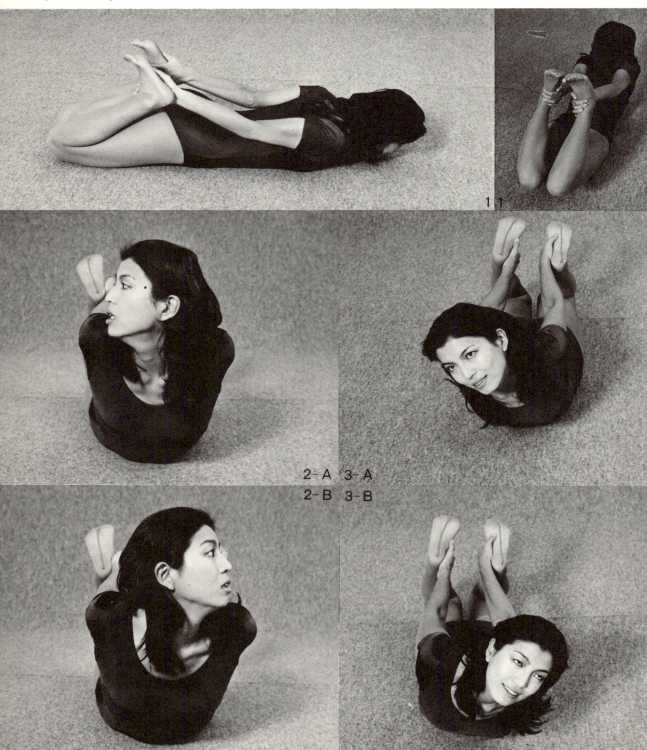

11

2-A 3-A
2-B 3-B

Movements and Breathing Order

1. Sitting on the floor with your legs spread wide, raise your right arm high over your head.

2. Inhaling then exhaling, bend and twist your body forward until your right hand extends well beyond the toes of your left foot.

3–4. Repeat with your left hand.

Effects

Extending the muscles of the undersides of your feet and of the lateral abdomen, this exercise corrects malplacement of internal organs and relieves congestion of the blood vessels and anemia. In addition, it improves the functioning of the ears.

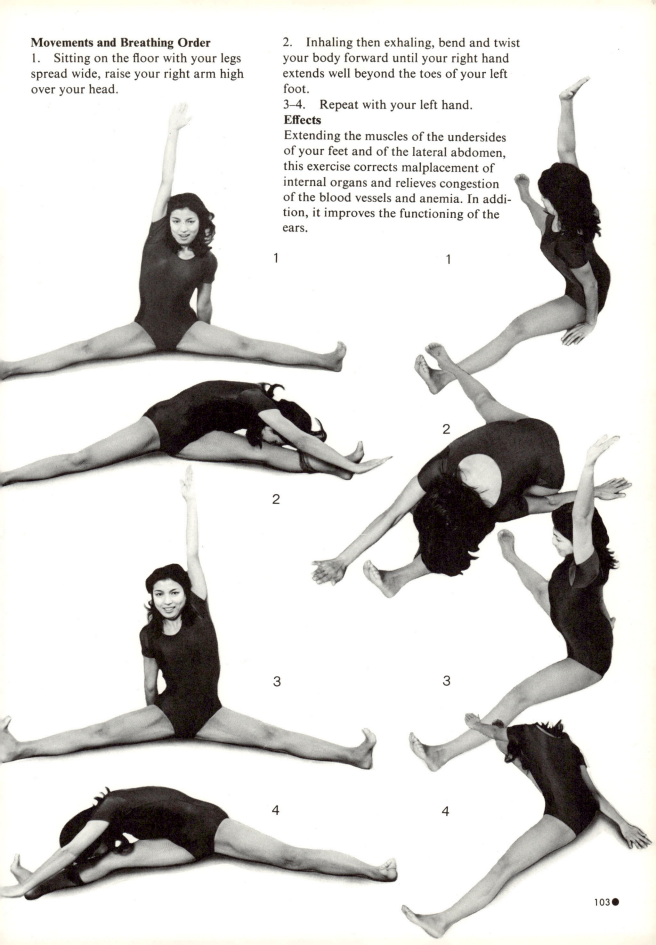

1

1

2

2

3

3

4

4

Movements and Breathing Order

1.   Kneeling upright with your toes pointed and your heels spread apart, press both sides of your nose with your index fingers.

2.   Rubbing upward with your fingers, inhale and, as you exhale, lean your upper body backward.

Effects

This exercise relieves congestion of the blood in the area of the chest and the sacral vertebrae and the nose.

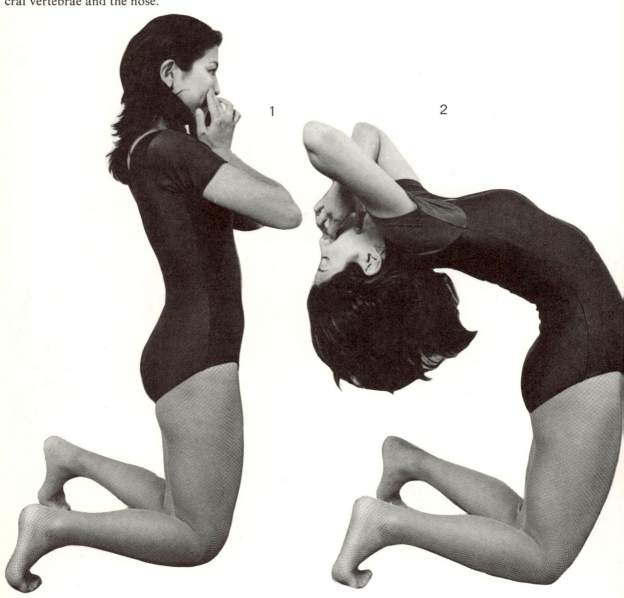

1

2

Stiffness in the Neck and Shoulders

Goals and Effects

Causes of stiffness in the neck and shoulders include psychological tension, organic abnormalities, irregularities in blood pressure, insufficient nourishment, poor posture, and muscular fatigue. Consequently, these exercises concentrate on limbering the neck and shoulders and strengthening the abdomen. To do this, they employ movements that relax the shoulders and cause forward extensions of both arms. Furthermore, because of the relations between them and the neck, the exercises employ movements that limber the wrists and ankles. Obstructions in the ankles cause slackening of the abdomen, tension in the shoulders, forward thrust of the chin, and twisted neck. For this reason, it is important always to tense the big toes, extend the Achilles' tendons, and keep the ankles in natural positions. Limbering the muscles of the neck and chest is of the greatest importance in eliminating contraction in those areas and thus in curing twisted neck. Applying stimulus to close sutures helps cure twisted neck resulting from sagging of the cranium.

Movements and Breathing Order

1.   Lying on your back, bend your arms at right angles upward beside your head. Hold your legs together, extend your Achilles' tendons and pull your chin in.

2.   Inhale and, as you exhale, raise both feet about thirty centimeters from the floor. Exhaling, lower them to a height of about five centimeters from the floor then, inhaling again, raise them to their former height. Repeat as you gradually spread your legs (3 and 4).

Effects

Since the chest in not relaxed, this exercise raises the body's balance center and thus relieves stiffness in the neck and shoulders. It further increases abdominal pressure to strengthen the muscles of the back. Gradually spreading the legs corrects troubles in the back and abdomen.

1
2

3
4

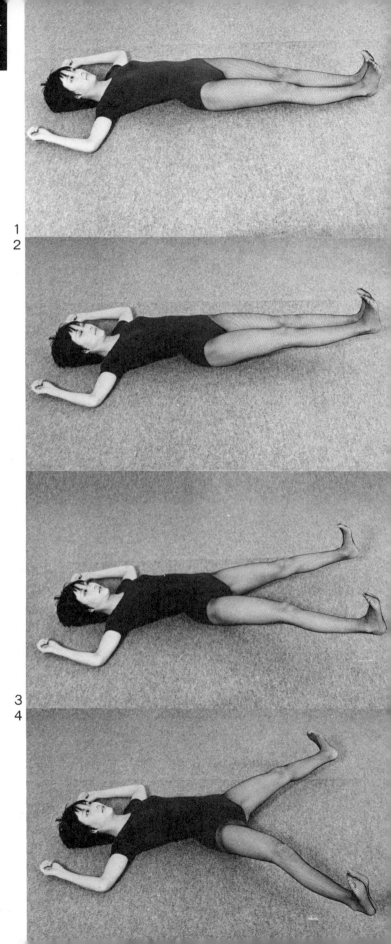

Movements and Breathing Order

Lying on your back, hold both arms at right angles pointed downward beside your body. Keeping both legs together, extend your Achilles' tendons and pull your chin in. Throughout the exercises, do not allow your fists to leave the floor.

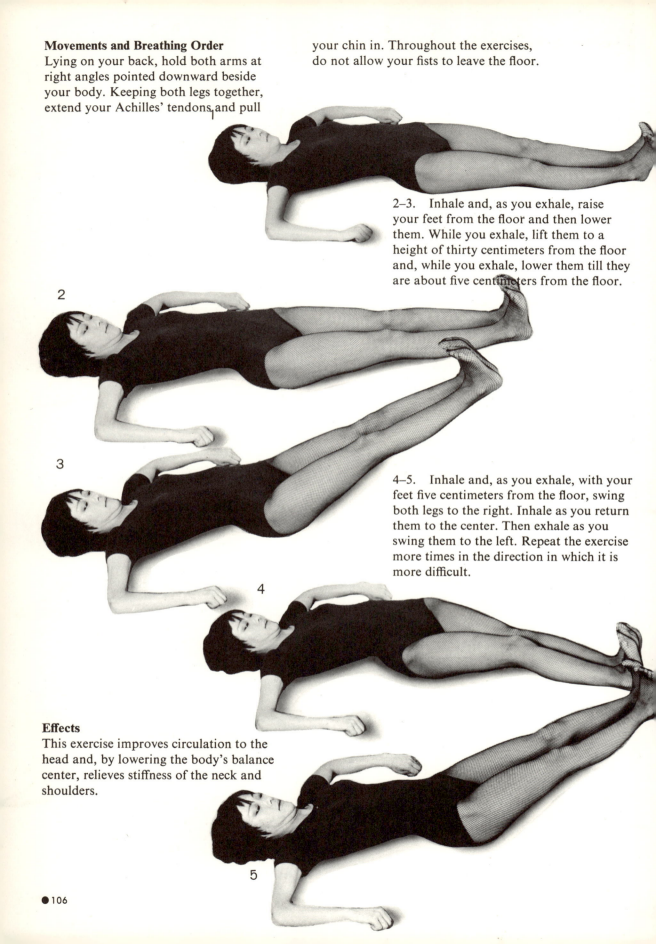

2–3.   Inhale and, as you exhale, raise your feet from the floor and then lower them. While you exhale, lift them to a height of thirty centimeters from the floor and, while you exhale, lower them till they are about five centimeters from the floor.

4–5.   Inhale and, as you exhale, with your feet five centimeters from the floor, swing both legs to the right. Inhale as you return them to the center. Then exhale as you swing them to the left. Repeat the exercise more times in the direction in which it is more difficult.

Effects

This exercise improves circulation to the head and, by lowering the body's balance center, relieves stiffness of the neck and shoulders.

Movements and Breathing Order

1. Lying on your back with your knees up, spread your feet about as far apart as your hips are wide and stretch both arms straight above your head.

2. Inhale and, as you exhale, raise your hips from the floor. Then raise your shoulders from the floor and stretch your arms as far above your head as possible. The upper part of your body should be supported by your head only. As you inhale, lower your body till your shoulders touch the floor. Repeat (1–3).

3–5. Then, when your upper body is supported on your head only, as you inhale, swing both arms round in a large circle until your hands reach your hips.

6–7. As you inhale, raise both arms and swing them from your hips upward toward your head again. At this time, your body should be bent so that your chin points up as in the position in step 3. Repeat this exercise.

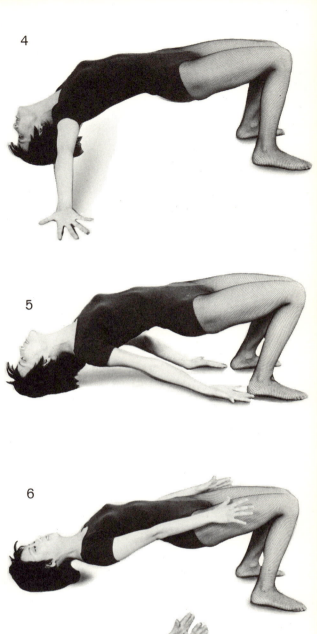

1

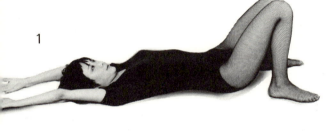

2

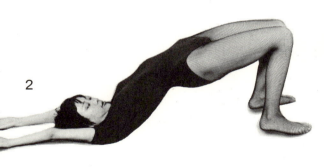

3

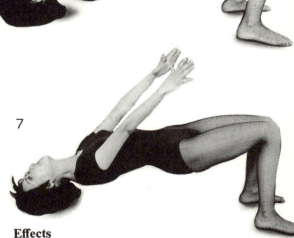

Effects
Raising and moving your hips forward and backward and swinging your arms relieve blood congestion in the shoulders.

Movements and Breathing Order

1. Lying on your back with your arms outstretched along both sides (palms down), tuck in your chin and extend your Achilles' tendons.

2–4. Inhale and, as you exhale, slowly raise your legs until your feet (toes only) touch the floor above your head.

5–6. Join the fingers of your hands and, inhaling then exhaling, further extend your left knee and left Achilles' tendon as you bring your right knee to a point beside your right ear.

7. Inhaling, relax your left knee and return your right foot and leg to their position in step 5. As you exhale, tense your right knee and right Achilles' tendon and bring your left knee to a point beside your left ear.

Effects

This exercise relieves congestion in the lower abdomen, corrects irregular organic sagging, strengthens the internal organs, and relieves stiffness in the neck and shoulders coming from them. In addition, by directly stimulating them, it relieves congestion in the shoulders and neck. It further relieves contraction in the back.

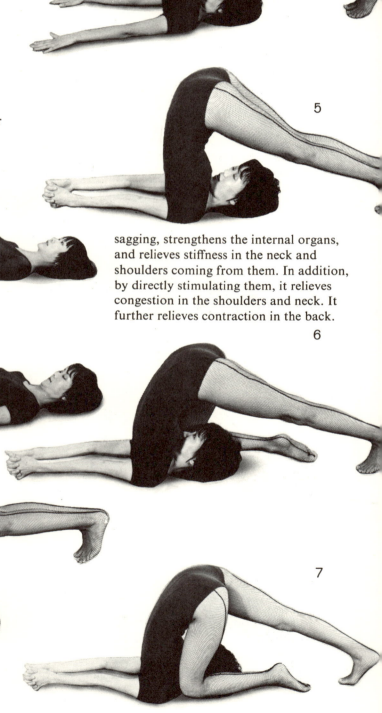

Movements and Breathing Order

1.   Lying on your stomach, spread your feet wide. Only your toes should be on the floor. Extend one arm over your head and one to the side.

2.   Inhale and, as you exhale, raise the arm stretched to the side toward the ceiling and twist your trunk.

3–4.   Without removing your feet from the floor, further twist your upper body until your raised arm describes a large circle and comes to the floor on the opposite side. As you inhale, return to the position in step 1. Then repeat with the other arm.

Effects

Twisting the body returns the internal organs to their normal positions and cures stiffness in the neck and shoulders resulting from irregular placement. This exercise further relieves stiffness in the upper back and the shoulder blades.

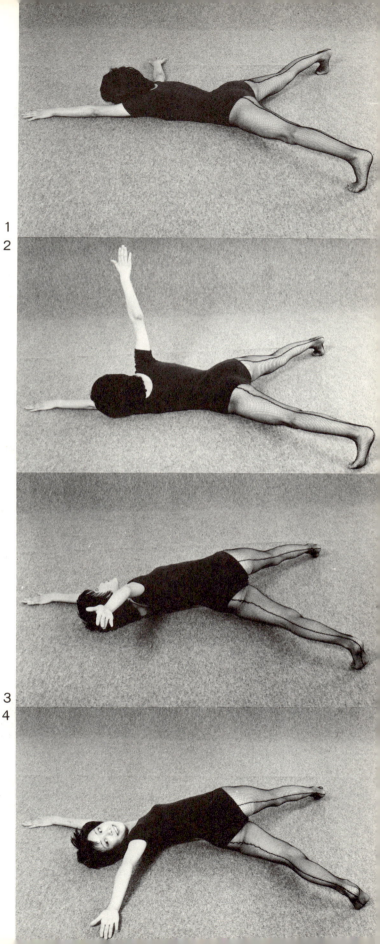

1

2

3

4

Movements and Breathing Order

1. Crouch on all fours so that your hands are about as far apart as your shoulders are wide and your knees about as far apart as your hips are wide.

2–3. Put your right shoulder on the floor in the position in which your left hand was and extend your right arm on the floor to the left side. Then join the palm of your left hand with that of your right one.

4–5. Inhale and, as you exhale, raise your left hand and arm upward in a large circle to the right until it touches the floor. As you inhale, return your left arm to the position in step 3. Repeat the exercise in the other direction.

Effects

This exercise corrects stiffness in the upper vertebrae by regulating the placement of the internal organs.

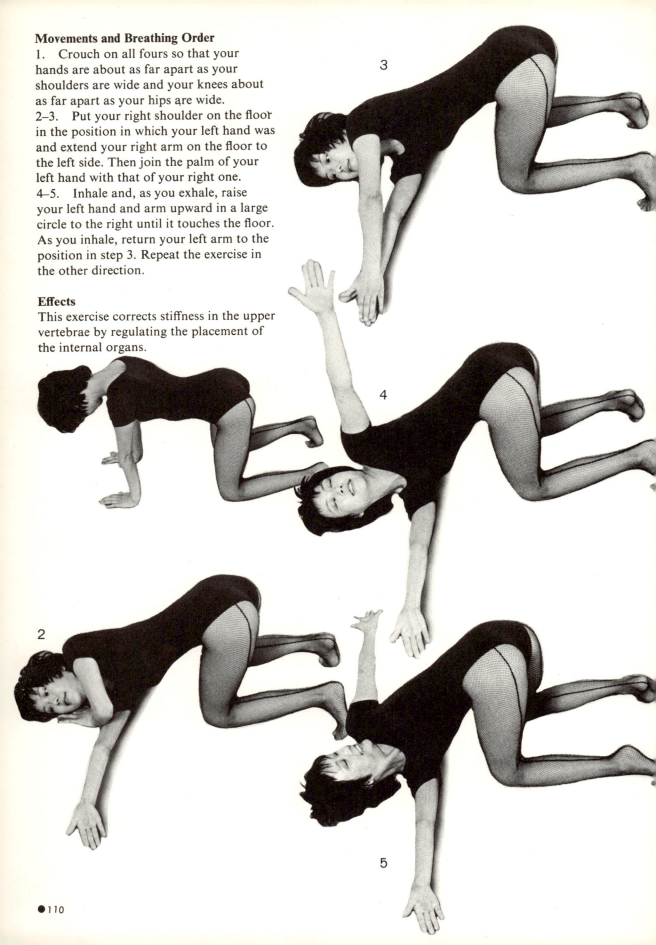

Movement and Breathing Order

1. Crouching on your knees, with only the toes of your feet on the floor, place the upper part of your forehead on the floor and put your hands on the floor to the sides of your head.

2. Inhale and, as you exhale, straighten your legs and raise your hips.

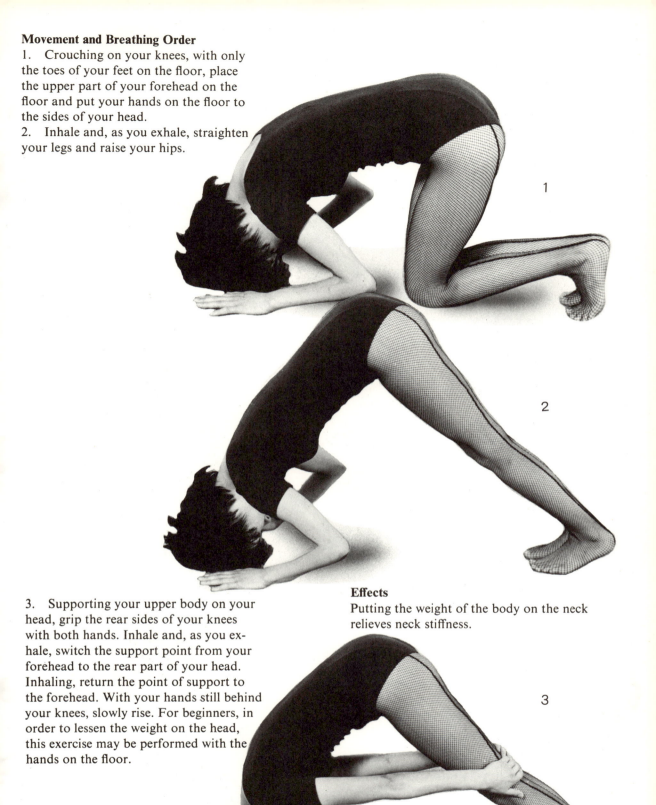

3. Supporting your upper body on your head, grip the rear sides of your knees with both hands. Inhale and, as you exhale, switch the support point from your forehead to the rear part of your head. Inhaling, return the point of support to the forehead. With your hands still behind your knees, slowly rise. For beginners, in order to lessen the weight on the head, this exercise may be performed with the hands on the floor.

Effects

Putting the weight of the body on the neck relieves neck stiffness.

Movements and Breathing Order

1. Kneeling in the *seiza* position, lock the fingers of both hands behind your back and, turning palms down, thrust your chest forward.

2. Inhale and, as you exhale, raise your hands in the direction of your head.

3–4. Continue raising your hands as you lean your trunk forward until your forehead touches the floor.

5–7. Inhale and, as you exhale, continue raising your hands and hips. Gradually roll forward so that the back part of your head rests on the floor. Inhaling, roll back until your forehead touches the floor.

Effects

Bending forward and putting your weight on your neck as you join your arms behind your back stimulates and relieves stiffness in the shoulders.

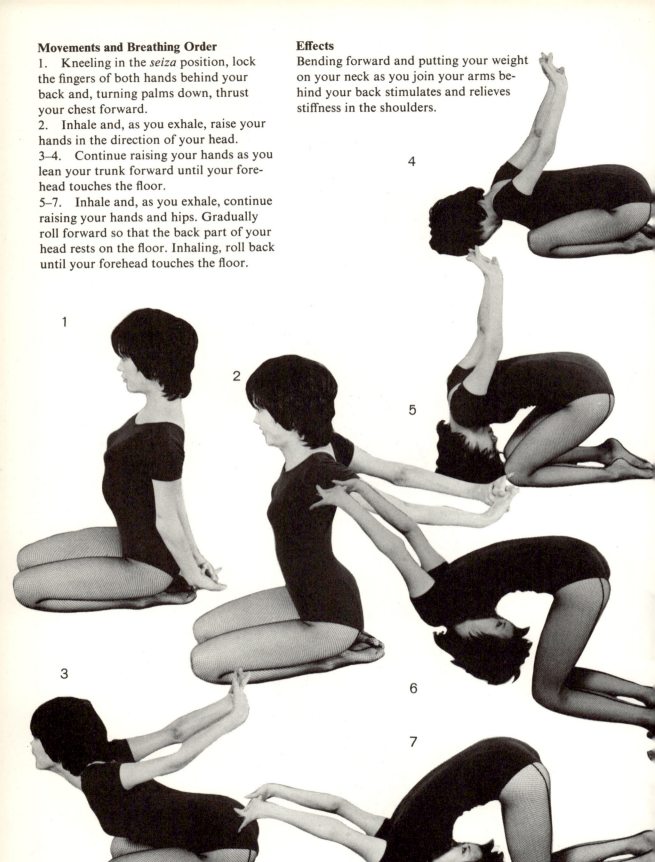

Movements and Breathing Order

1. Sitting on the floor with legs straight in front of you, extend your Achilles' tendons and neck. Behind your back, grip one wrist in the fingers of the other hand.

2–3. Inhale and, as you exhale, turn your neck to the left while raising your hands high behind you.

4. Inhale and, as you exhale, turn your neck still further and raise your hands still further. Lean forward. Then repeat in the opposite direction.

Effects

Twisting your neck and bending forward extends the muscles of the neck. Joining your hands behind your back relieves stiffness in the shoulders. Leaning forward increases abdominal pressure and relieves both constipation and the shoulder and neck stiffness resulting from it.

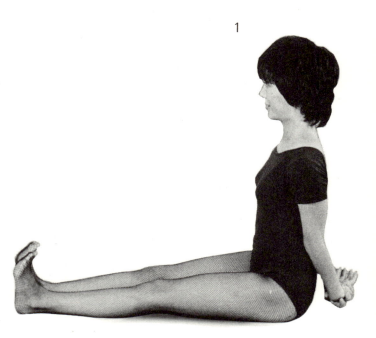

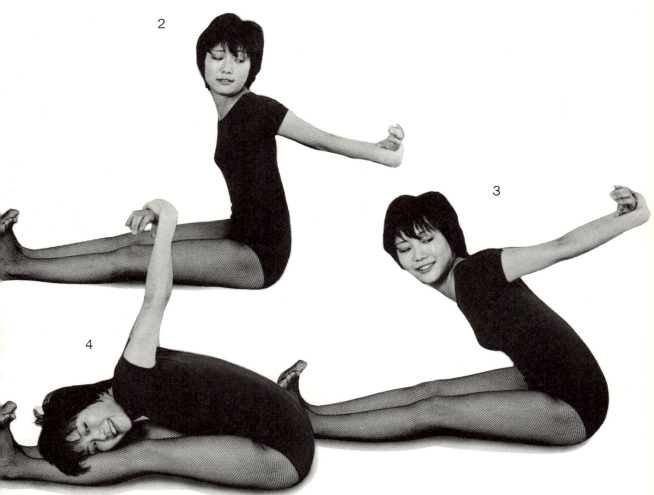

Asthma

Goals and Effects

Irregularities in body secretions stimulate paralysis of the respiratory organs in the sickness that is known as asthma. These irregularities can arise from abnormalities in the nervous, endocrine, or metabolic systems. The coughing itself is not the sickness: it is the body's way of trying to cure the trouble. Consequently, it is dangerous to attempt to suppress the cough. Congestion in the chest and above reduces the volume of intake of breath and the volume of gases exhaled. Since the aims of exercises for the cure of asthma are to relieve contraction and congestion in the neck and chest and to concentrate strength in the hip and abdomen region, they involve actions that expand the chest, stretch the neck, expand the iliac bone, extend the side muscles, and limber the muscles of the arms and legs.

These movements stimulate the operation of the vagus nerve and suppress abnormal excitement of the sympathetic nervous system. In addition, they relieve blood congestion in the abdomen and chest and thus strengthen and stimulate the functioning of the lungs and heart.

Movements and Breathing Order

1. Lying on your stomach with both legs together and outstretched rearward, extend both arms and hands (palms down) on the floor above your head and regulate your breathing.
2. With both hands together and with fingers turned back to form a forty-five-degree angle with your wrists, raise both hands to expand your chest fully. Keep your eyes on your fingertips. Inhaling, return your body to the position in step 1 and regulate your breathing.
3. Inhale and, as you exhale, without bending your knees, stretch your body and raise your legs from the thighs. Inhaling, return your body to the position in step 1.

Effects

This exercise relieves congestion in the chest and abdomen and promotes natural breathing by eliminating contraction of the ribs.

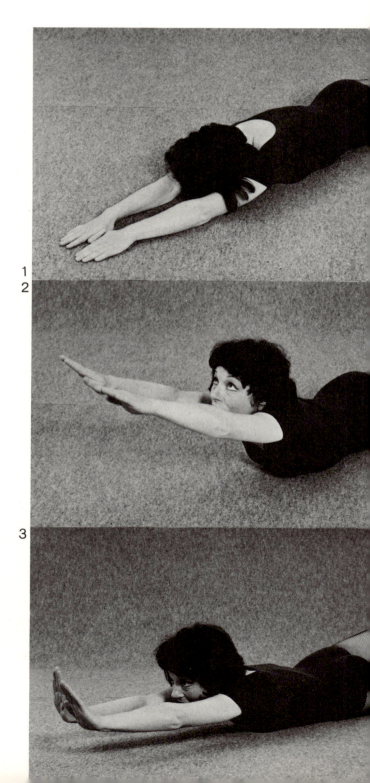

Movements and Breathing Order

1. Lying on your back, join your hands behind your neck. Your elbows must be on the floor. With your legs outstretched straight, extend your Achilles' tendons and pull your chin in, as you regulate your breathing.

2. Keeping them together, bend your knees. Inhaling then exhaling, raise your feet about ten centimeters from the floor.

Hold them in this position. Then inhale and, as you exhale, slowly lower your feet.

Effects

This exercise relieves contraction and congestion in the chest and thoracic area. In addition, it lowers the body's center of balance by concentrating strength in the hips and abdomen.

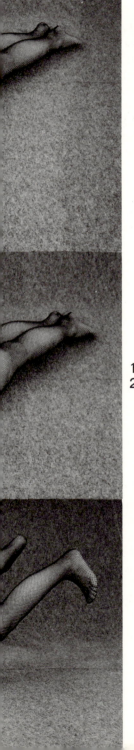

1
2

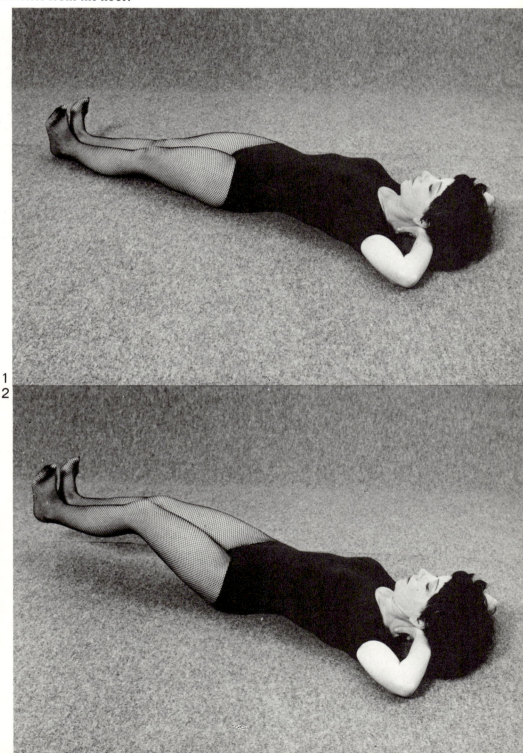

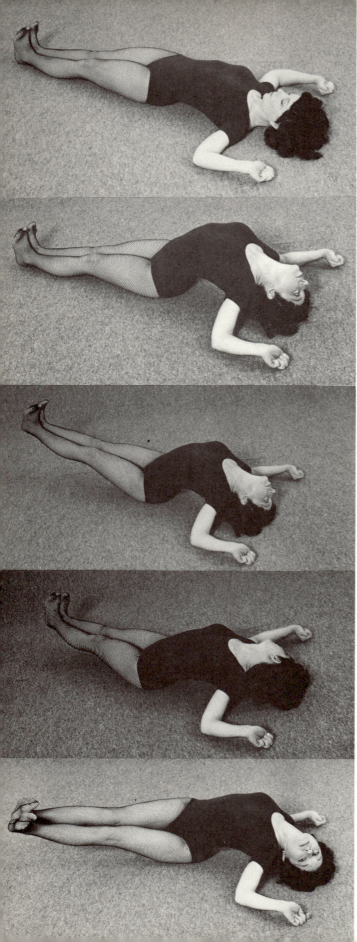

1
2

3
4

5

Movements and Breathing Order

1. Lying on your back with legs outstretched and Achilles' tendons extended, put both arms on the floor bent at right angles upward beside your head and regulate your breathing.

2. Inhale and, as you exhale, without raising your knees from the floor, thrust your chin forward and, with your upper body resting on your head, raise your chest high.

3. Inhale and, as you exhale, extend your Achilles' tendons and raise your feet thirty centimeters from the floor.

4. Inhale and, as you exhale, turn your neck to the right. With your feet in the same position, twist your legs to the right from the thigh joints. Inhale as you return your legs and head to the central position.

5. Repeat, twisting to the left.

Effects

Raising your legs lowers the body's center of balance and relieves tension in the chest. Raising the arms in an L-shape as you lift your chest relieves contraction in the chest.

Movements and Breathing Order ▶

1. Lying on your back with your legs together and your Achilles' tendons extended, clench your fists (thumbs inside) and put your elbows on the floor at your sides. Raise your chest, thrust your chin out, and regulate your breathing.

2. Inhale and, as you exhale, raise and lower your legs in time with your breathing.

Effects

Arching your body in this way relieves blood congestion in the chest; and raising and lowering your legs strengthen your abdominal muscles.

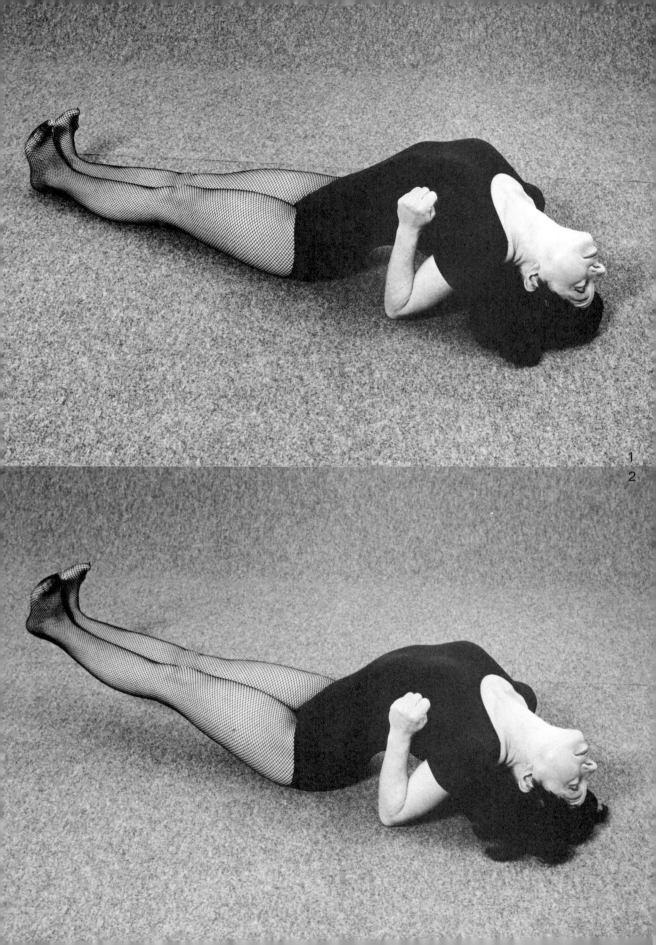

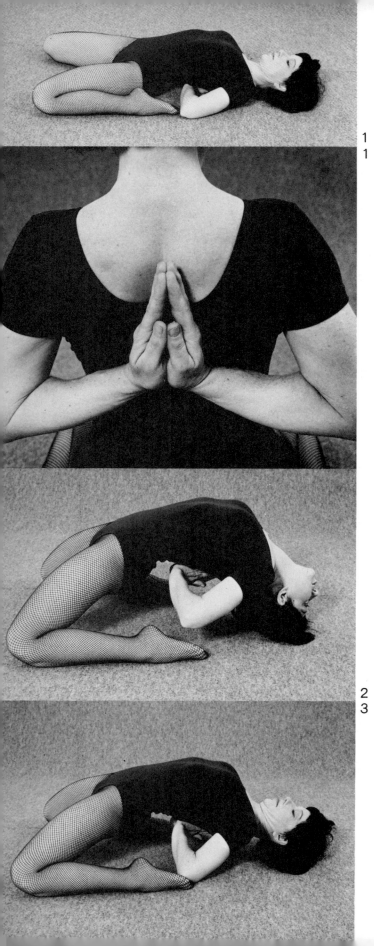

Movements and Breathing Order

1. Kneeling in the *seiza* position, spread your feet and lower your buttocks to the floor between them (*wariza*). Then, with your hands joined in the prayer attitude behind your back, lean over backward until you are lying face up on the floor. Regulate your breathing.

2. Inhale and, as you exhale, raise your chest high and thrust your chin out.

3. Inhale and relax your chest. Exhale and thrust your chest upward. Breathe rhythmically as you do this.

Effects

This exercise regulates the pelvis and stimulates the chest, which is related to the pelvis. Holding your hands behind your back in this way as you raise your chest relieves contraction in both the hands and the chest.

Movements and Breathing Order ▶

1. Lying on your back, pull your knees to your chest with both arms. Regulate your breathing.

2. Inhale and, as you exhale, pull your chin inward, raise your head off the floor, and pull your knees still closer to your chest. Without releasing your legs, inhale as you relax your arms and neck. Repeat several times.

Effects

This exercise lowers the pubic bone and regulates the pelvis and in this way regulates the ribs, which are related to these parts of the body.

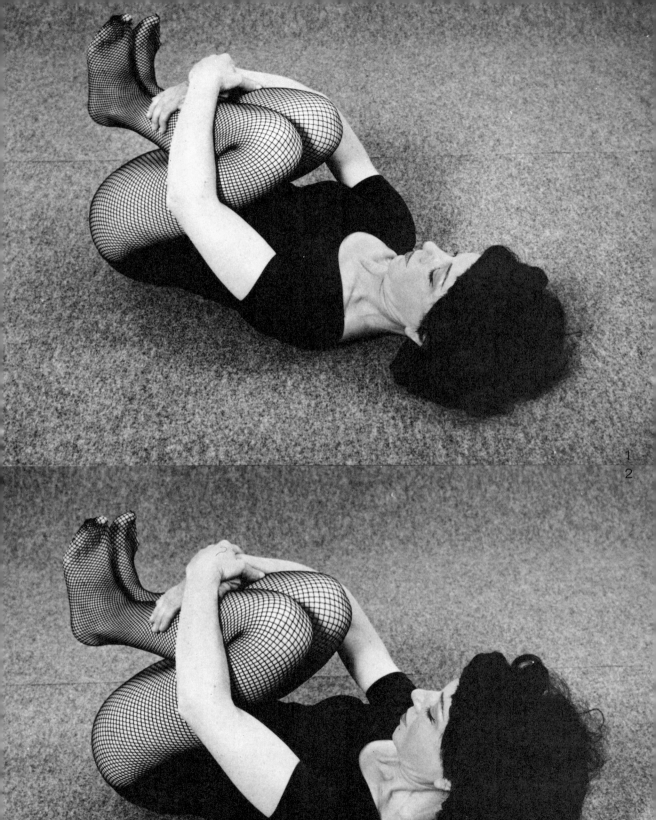

Movements and Breathing Order

1. Put your toes on a box or something high enough to allow you to hold your body parallel with the floor when you stand on your arms in the way shown in the photograph. Bend your back slightly and look forward.

2. From this position, inhale and, as you exhale, do several pushups.

3. Change the direction in which your hands are turned—from forward to out- ward, inward, and rearward (A and B). When you point them to the rear, place your hands slightly rearward.

Effects

Power of the arms is comparable to breathing power and to the ability of the rib cage to open and close. Because it calls for changing the direction of the hands, this exercise has a total improving effect on respiration.

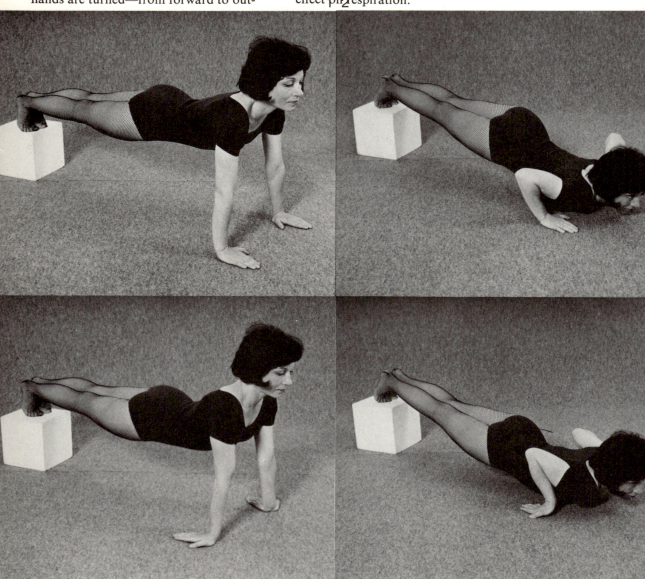

3-A   3-B

Movements and Breathing Order

1–2. Sitting on the floor with your legs outstretched in front of you and your Achilles' tendons extended, join both hands behind your back and outstretch your arms. Expand your chest as you raise your arms high.

3. Inhale and, as you exhale, expand your chest further and lean forward.

4. Inhale and, as you exhale, turn your body to the right.

5. Inhale and return your body to the front. Exhaling, twist your upper body in the opposite direction.

Effects

This exercise relieves contraction in the hands, shoulder blades, and undersides of the feet.

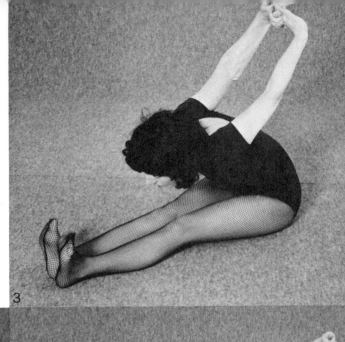

3

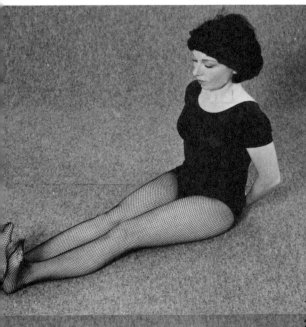

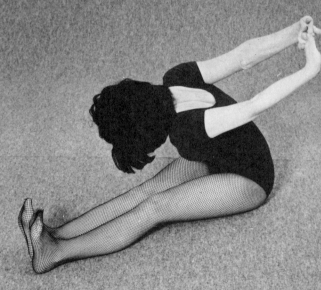

1 4
2 5

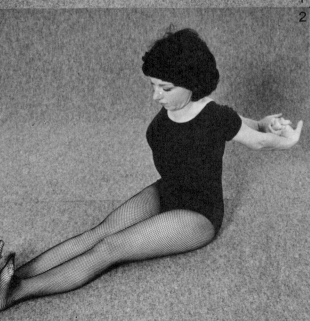

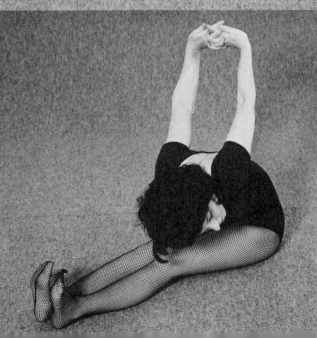

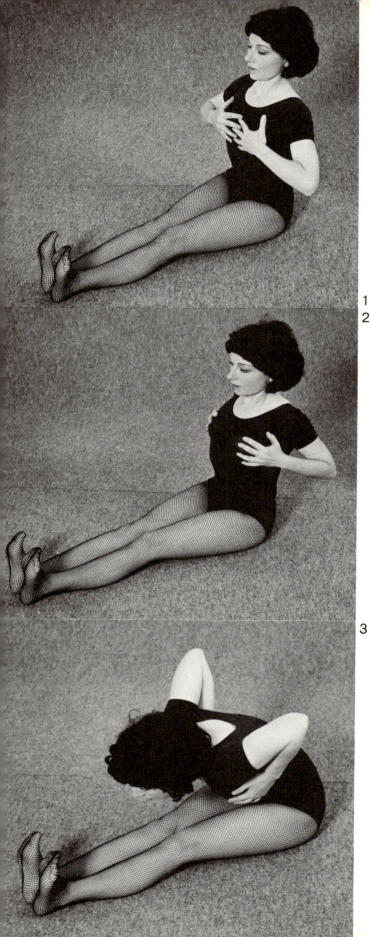

Movements and Breathing Order

1–2. Sitting with your legs outstretched in front of you and with your Achilles' tendons extended, stretch your spine and pull your chin inward. Bring both hands to your chest.

3. Inhale and, exhaling, lean your trunk forward. Repeat, putting your hands first on the upper then on the middle and lower parts of your chest.

Effects

This exercise relieves contraction in the muscles of the chest and the undersides of the feet.

1
2

3

Strengthening the Interior Organs

Goals and Effects

Since the spinal cord is vitally important to the proper functioning of the liver, kidneys, and stomach—fourth and eighth thoracic vertebrae for the liver; fifth, sixth, and eleventh thoracic vertebrae for the stomach; and the tenth thoracic vertebra for the kidneys—good back carriage is of the utmost significance. Consequently, all of the exercises designed to treat illness in these organs pay special attention to limbering and strengthening the muscles of the hip and abdomen regions, to building up abdominal pressure, to improving circulation in the hips and abdomen, to correcting poor posture, and to stimulating and improving the functioning of the nervous system.

Movements and Breathing Order

1. Lying on your back, bend your knees and put your hands behind your neck.
2. Inhale and, as you exhale, lower your knees to the right. At the same time, turn your face to the left. Inhaling, return to the position in step 1.
3. As you exhale, lower your knees to the left and turn your face to the right. Inhaling, return to the position in step 1.
4–6. With your hands in the same position, raise your feet from the floor with knees bent so that your thighs are perfectly vertical. Repeat the movements of steps 1 through 3.
7–9. Next, with your hands in the same position, pull your thighs as close to your chest as possible and repeat the movements in steps 1 through 3.

Effects

Lowering your knees to the floor relieves blood congestion in the sides of the abdomen and improves the functioning of liver, kidneys, and stomach.

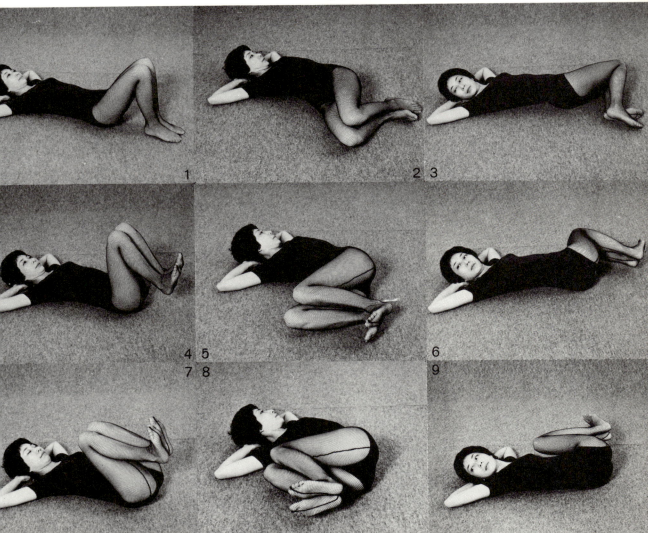

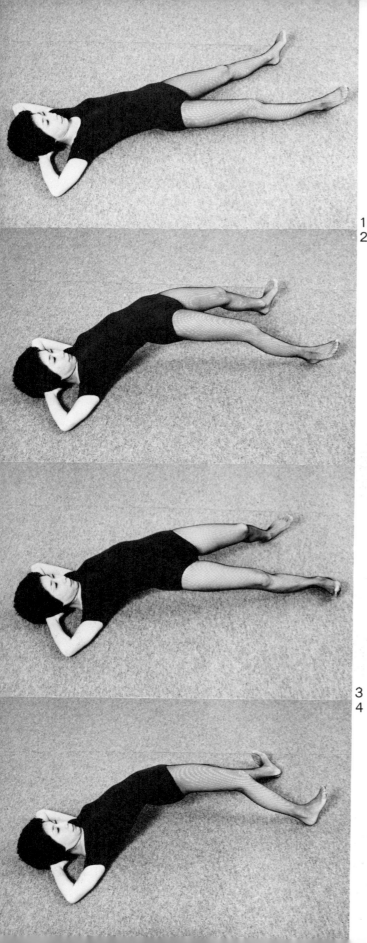

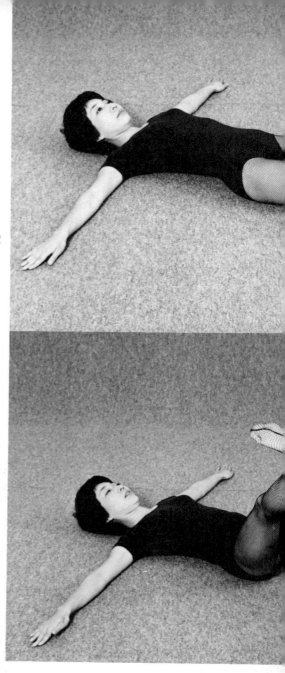

1
2

3
4

Movements and Breathing Order

1. Lying on your back, join both hands behind your neck and spread your feet to hip width.

2. Inhale and, as you exhale, raise your hips.

3. Inhale and, as you exhale, raise your hips still further and twist them to the right.

4. Raise your hips still further but twist them to the left. As you exhale, slowly lower your hips to the floor.

Effects

Raising and twisting your hips improve intestinal peristalsis and relieve blood congestion in the abdomen.

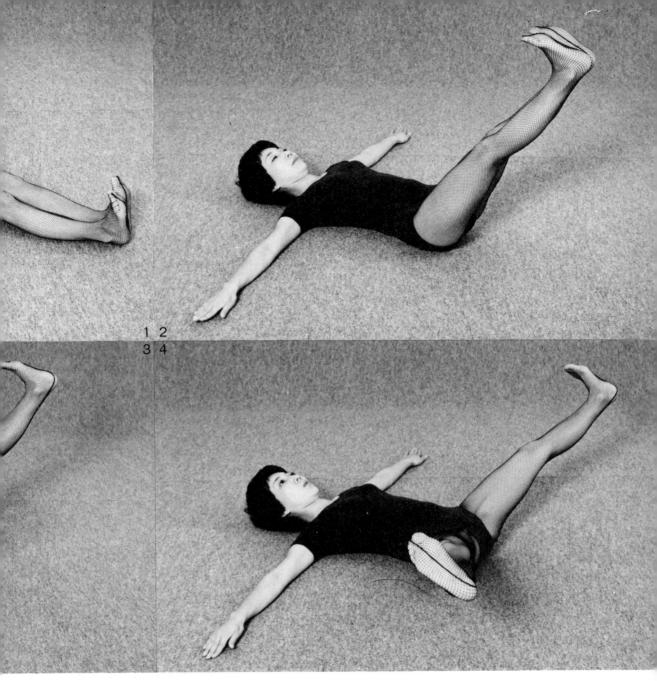

Movements and Breathing Order

1. Lying on your back, outstretch both arms straight to the sides at shoulder height. Holding your legs and feet together, tense your Achilles' tendons.

2. Inhale and, as you exhale, raise both legs together until they form an angle of forty-five degrees with the floor.

3. Inhale and, as you exhale, turn your feet inward.

4. Inhale, and as you exhale, turn both feet outward again. Slowly lower your legs to the floor.

Effects

Raising your legs in this way increases abdominal pressure and prevents sagging in the internal organs. Turning the legs inward and outward corrects balance in the placement of the organs.

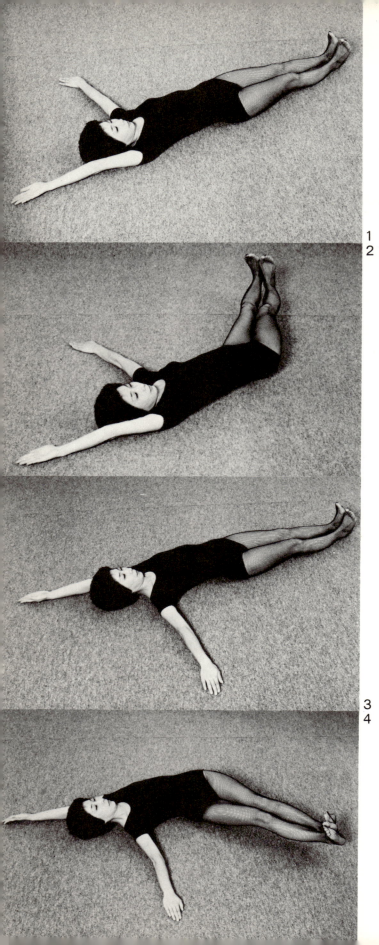

Movements and Breathing Order

1. Lying on your back with your legs together, stretch your left arm straight to the side and your right arm straight above your head.

2. Inhale and, as you exhale, swing both legs together to the left. Then raise and lower them. Raise them as you inhale and lower them as you exhale.

3–4. Stretching your right arm to the side and your left arm straight above your head, swing both legs together to the right. Raise and lower them in the fashion described in step 1. Slowly return them to the original position.

Effects

This exercise relieves contraction on the side of the raised arm and eliminates blood congestion. Raising and lowering the legs improve internal peristalsis.

Movements and Breathing Order ▶

1. Lying on your back, place both hands on your abdomen. Outstretch your right leg and bend your left leg, bringing your left foot to your right knee.

2–3. Inhale and, as you exhale, press or rub (upward) your abdomen. Raise your trunk from the floor at the same time. Repeat with the legs in reverse positions. Perform this exercise a number of times.

Effects

This exercise prevents overall sagging of the internal organs, relieves blood congestion in the abdomen, and increases abdominal pressure.

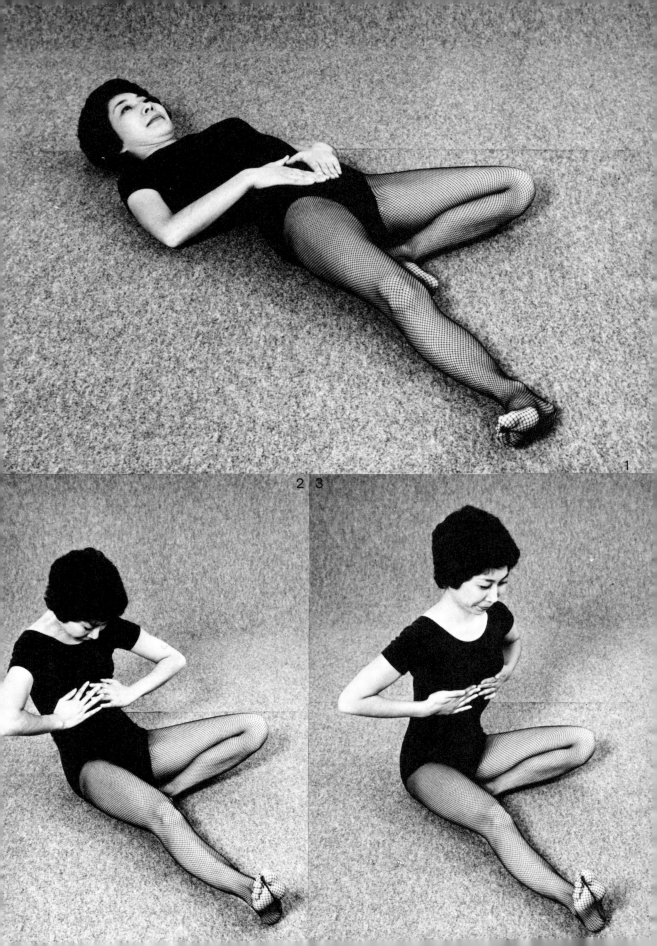

Movements and Breathing Order

1. Lying on your back, put both hands above your liver. Bend your right leg so that your right foot comes to your hips.

2–3. Inhale and, as you exhale, pressing on the part of your body above your liver, raise your trunk. Do not let your right knee leave the floor.

4–6. Press both hands against the area above your stomach. Repeat the movements in steps 2 and 3. Repeat several times, first with the left leg bent and then with the right leg bent.

Effects

The functioning of the organ above which you press your hands is improved by this exercise.

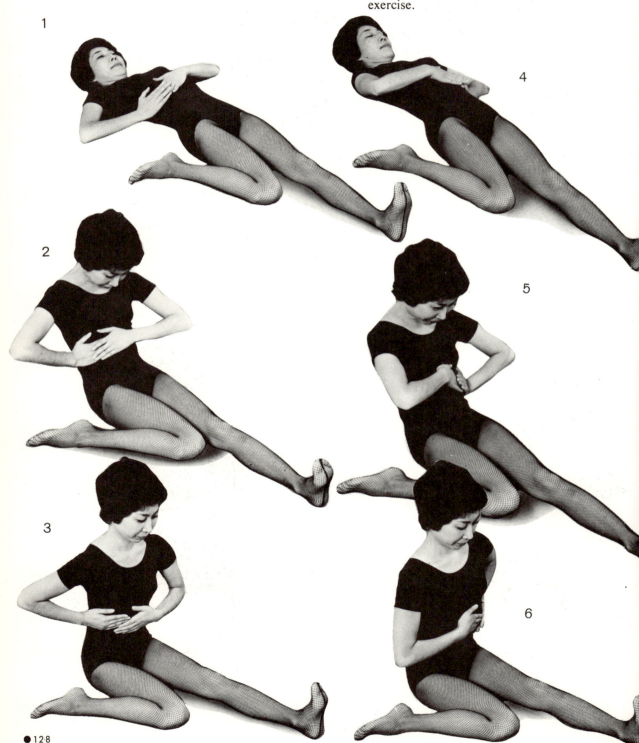

Movements and Breathing Order

1. Lie on your back in the *wariza* position (see p. 81) with both arms outstretched above your head.

2–3. Inhale and, as you exhale, twisting your hands inward, lift your trunk off the floor. Do not employ bouncing motions to do this and do not allow your knees to leave the floor.

Effects

Because of the maximum stimulation this exercise has on the hips and abdomen, it strengthens the diaphragm and vitalizes the functioning of the internal organs.

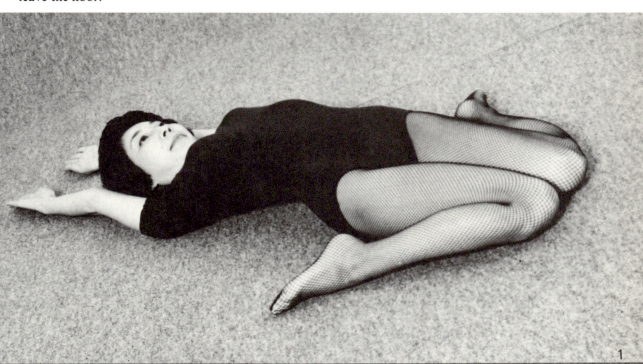

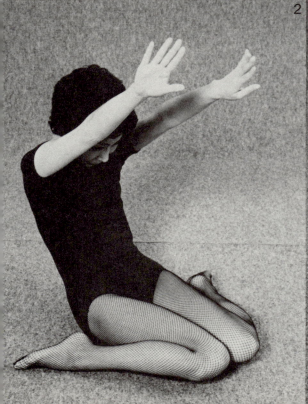

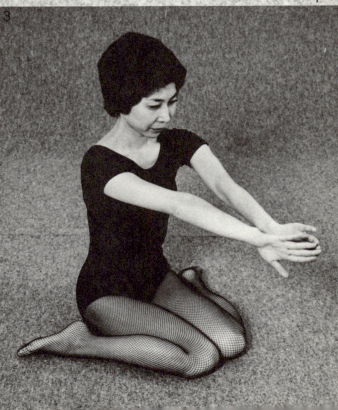

Movements and Breathing Order

1. Lying on your stomach, hands under your shoulders, raise your body until it is supported by toes and fingers only.
2. Inhale and, as you exhale, bend your elbows. As you inhale, straighten them again. Repeat several times.
4–5. Inhale and, as you exhale, twist your hips and lower your heels to the right side. At this time, look in the direction in which you have lowered your heels. After returning to the starting position, lower your heels to the left.

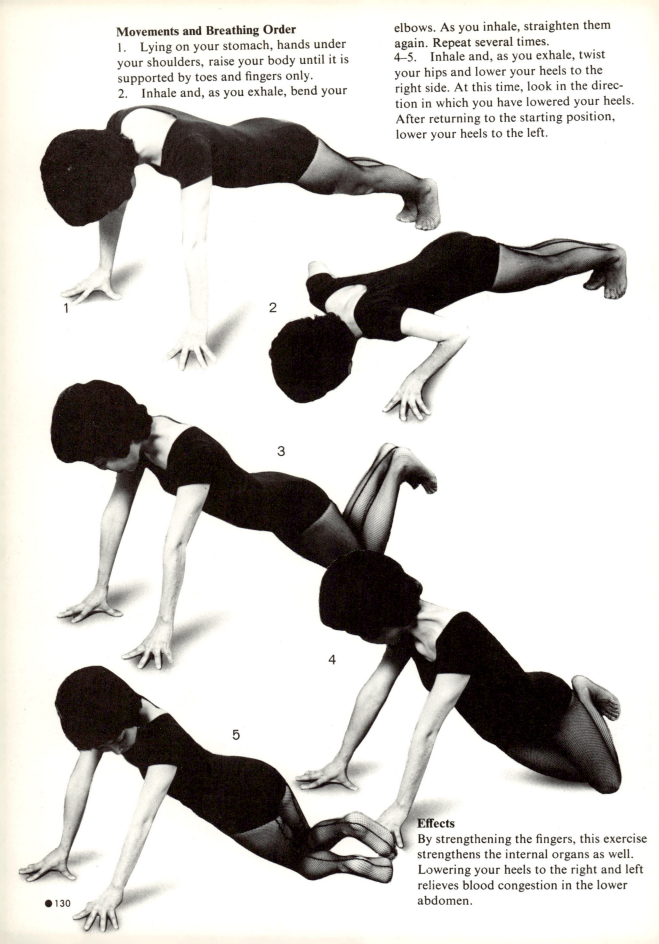

Effects

By strengthening the fingers, this exercise strengthens the internal organs as well. Lowering your heels to the right and left relieves blood congestion in the lower abdomen.

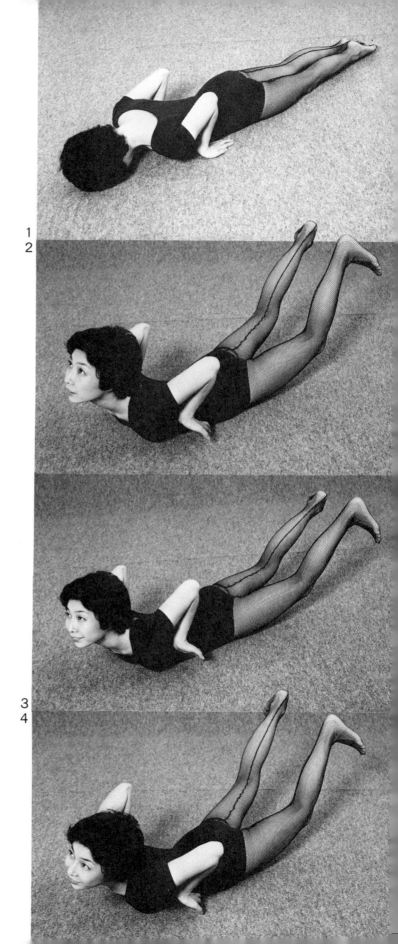

Movements and Breathing Order

1.   Lying on your stomach, with your hands—fingers pointed toward your feet—flat on the floor at your sides, extend both legs fully.

2.   Inhale and, as you exhale, raise your head and bend your trunk backward. Lift both hands and feet from the floor.

3–4.   Inhale and, as you exhale, bend both legs to the left and then to the right.

Effects

By extending the chest and abdominal muscles, this exercise stimulates circulation to the heart and improves both digestion and elimination.

Movements and Breathing Order

1. Lying on your stomach, put your left hand in the small of your back and your right hand behind your head.
2. Inhale and, as you exhale, raise your trunk from the floor.
3. Inhale and, as you exhale, twist your trunk to the left. Inhaling, return to the starting position.
4–6. This time, with your right hand in the small of your back and your left hand behind your head, repeat, twisting your trunk to the right.

Effects

Twisting your trunk relieves contraction on the opposite side of the body. Since this stimulates the sacral vertebrae, it improves peristalsis in the lower abdomen.

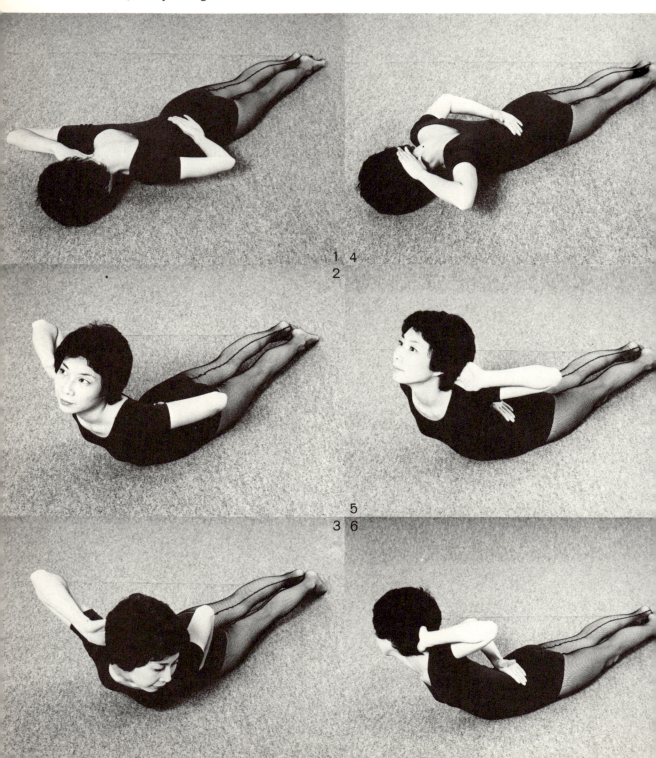

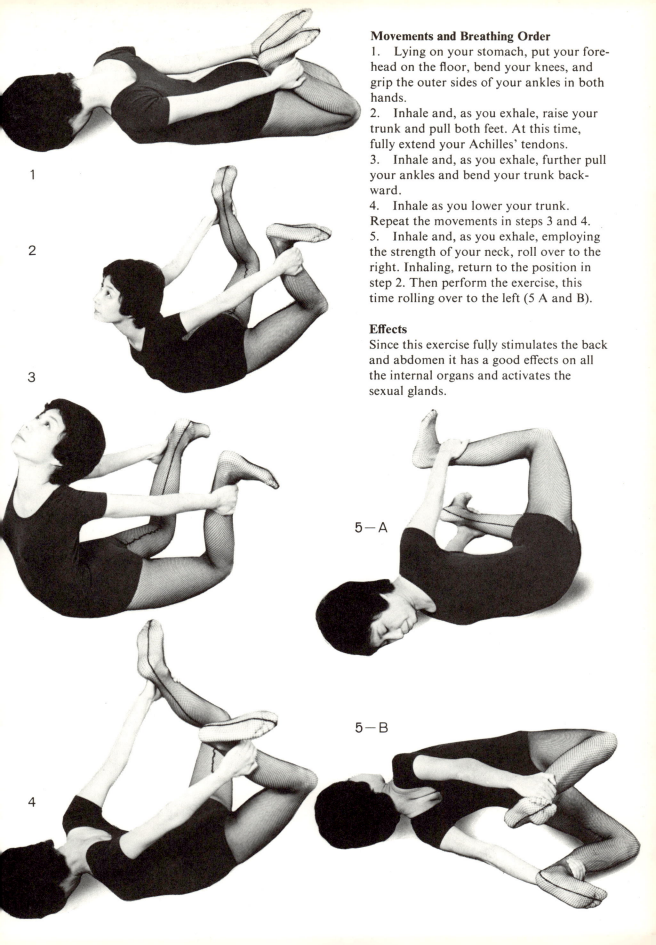

1

2

3

4

Movements and Breathing Order

1. Lying on your stomach, put your forehead on the floor, bend your knees, and grip the outer sides of your ankles in both hands.

2. Inhale and, as you exhale, raise your trunk and pull both feet. At this time, fully extend your Achilles' tendons.

3. Inhale and, as you exhale, further pull your ankles and bend your trunk backward.

4. Inhale as you lower your trunk. Repeat the movements in steps 3 and 4.

5. Inhale and, as you exhale, employing the strength of your neck, roll over to the right. Inhaling, return to the position in step 2. Then perform the exercise, this time rolling over to the left (5 A and B).

Effects

Since this exercise fully stimulates the back and abdomen it has a good effects on all the internal organs and activates the sexual glands.

5 — A

5 — B

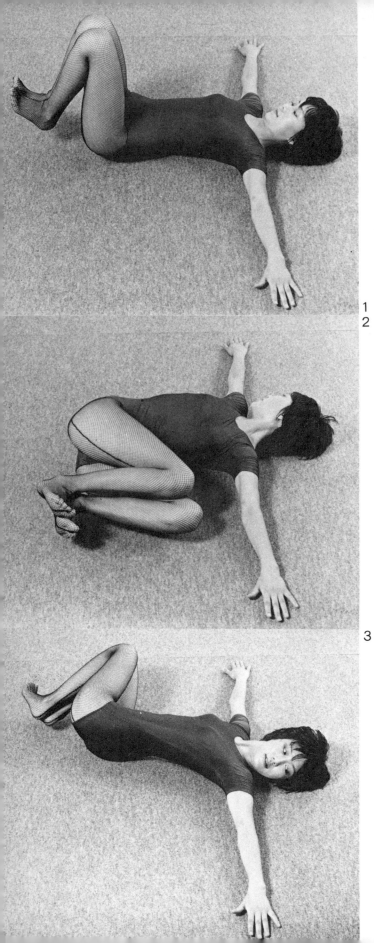

1
2

3

Sagging of the Internal Organs

Goals and Effects

Unless the organs are in their natural positions, poor circulation, insufficient nourishment, and general bad health result. But since sagging of the organs is caused by an overall sagging of the whole body, medicines will not cure it. People with this kind of constitution have weak abdomens and arms, the muscles of the undersides of their feet are contracted, and they put their weight on the outer sides of their feet. Curing the condition entails rectifying these faults.

The exercises shown here strengthen the muscles of the hips and abdomen and the pelvis and in this way improve circulation to the internal organs. In addition, they relax the shoulders and neck while increasing tension in the organs and correcting the placement of the musculature and generally improving the physique.

Movements and Breathing Order

1. Lying on your back, outstretch both arms to your sides, bend your knees, tense your Achilles' tendons, and raise your feet from the floor.
2. As you exhale, lower both knees to the left and turn your face to the right. As you inhale, return to the position in step 1.
3. As you exhale, lower both knees to the right and turn your face to the left. Inhale as you return to the position in step 1. Repeat several times.

Effects

Bending your legs and twisting your hips correct abnormal placement of the internal organs.

Movements and Breathing Order ▶

1–2. Lying on your back with both hands interlocked high above your head. Bend your knees and, exhaling, lift your hips from the floor. Suddenly relax and lower your hips without allowing them to touch the floor. Then lift them again. Repeat several times.

Effects

Since this exercise increases abdominal pressure and strengthens the internal organs, it corrects organic placement naturally.

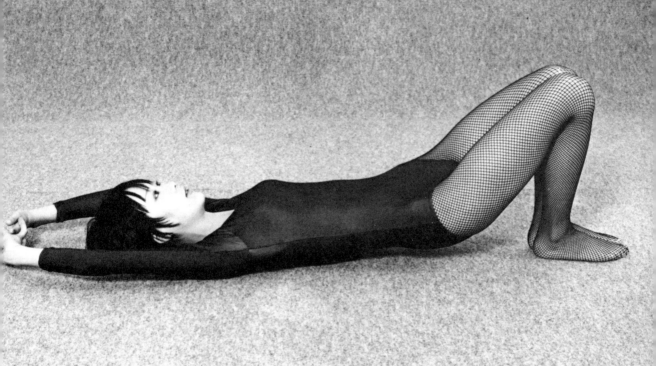

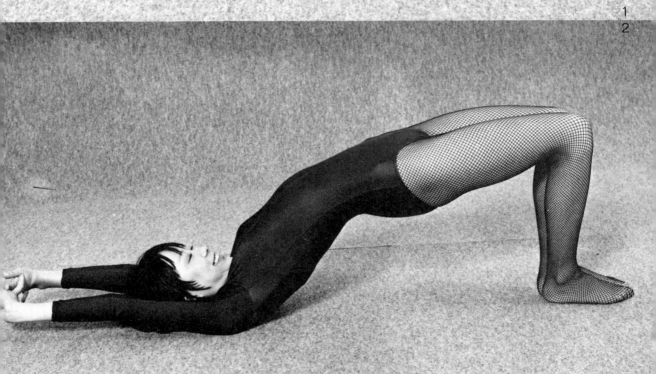

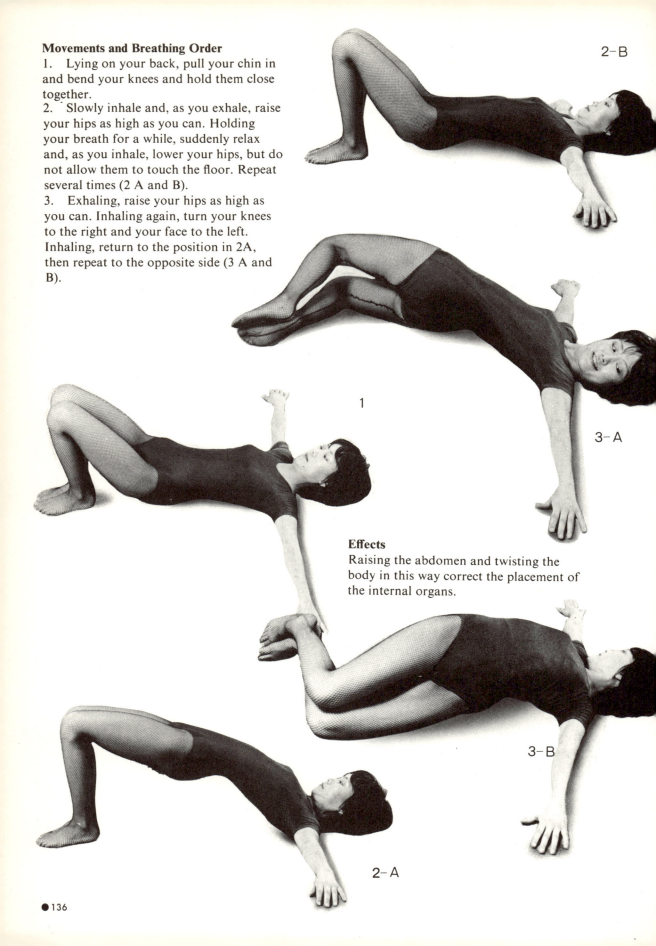

Movements and Breathing Order

1.   Lying on your back, pull your chin in and bend your knees and hold them close together.

2.   Slowly inhale and, as you exhale, raise your hips as high as you can. Holding your breath for a while, suddenly relax and, as you inhale, lower your hips, but do not allow them to touch the floor. Repeat several times (2 A and B).

3.   Exhaling, raise your hips as high as you can. Inhaling again, turn your knees to the right and your face to the left. Inhaling, return to the position in 2A, then repeat to the opposite side (3 A and B).

2–B

1

3–A

Effects
Raising the abdomen and twisting the body in this way correct the placement of the internal organs.

3–B

2–A

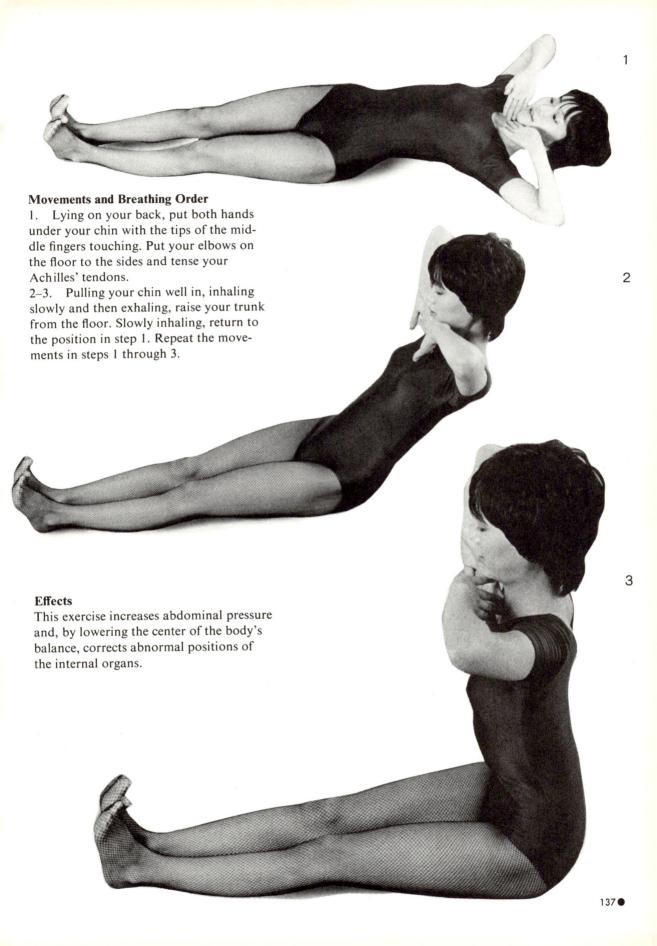

Movements and Breathing Order

1.   Lying on your back, put both hands under your chin with the tips of the middle fingers touching. Put your elbows on the floor to the sides and tense your Achilles' tendons.

2–3.   Pulling your chin well in, inhaling slowly and then exhaling, raise your trunk from the floor. Slowly inhaling, return to the position in step 1. Repeat the movements in steps 1 through 3.

Effects

This exercise increases abdominal pressure and, by lowering the center of the body's balance, corrects abnormal positions of the internal organs.

137

Movements and Breathing Order

1. Lying on your back, place your hands at the lower border of your rib cage and tense your Achilles' tendons.

2. Inhale and, as you exhale, raise your chest. Keep your Achilles' tendons tense and have the feeling that you are trying to press your shoulder blades against the lower part of your back.

3. With your toes together, raise your feet thirty centimeters off the floor. Ex-haling, lower them without letting them reach the floor. Repeat several times.

Effects

This fish pose corrects sagging of the ribs and the resulting displacement of the internal organs. Tensing the abdomen increases abdominal pressure, strengthens the hips, and corrects placement of the internal organs.

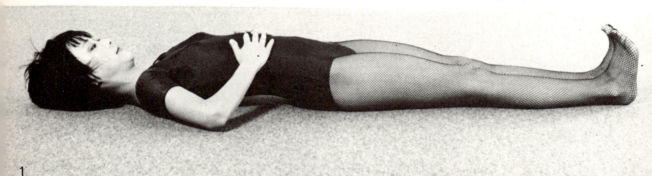

1

2

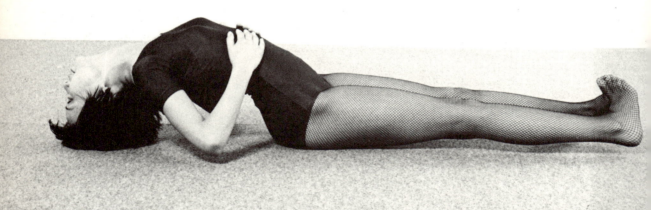

3

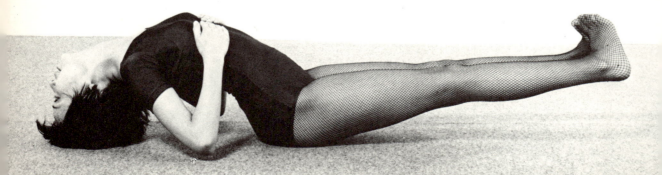

Movements and Breathing Order

1. Lying on your back with your arms—elbows bent—to the sides of your head, put the heel of your right foot on the toes of your left foot. Tense the Achilles' tendons of both feet and do not allow your elbows to leave the floor throughout the exercise.

2. Exhaling, thrust your chest upward and raise your trunk, turning your head backward.

3. In this position, inhaling then exhaling, raise and lower your feet. Exhale as you raise them and inhale as you lower them. Repeat, breathing rhythmically and placing special stress on exhaling forcefully. In a similar fashion, in the position in step 3, swing your legs to the right and left.

Effects

This exercise corrects forward stoops and relieves blood congestion in the chest. Raising and lowering and swinging the legs from side to side correct malplacement of the internal organs and invigorate peristalsis.

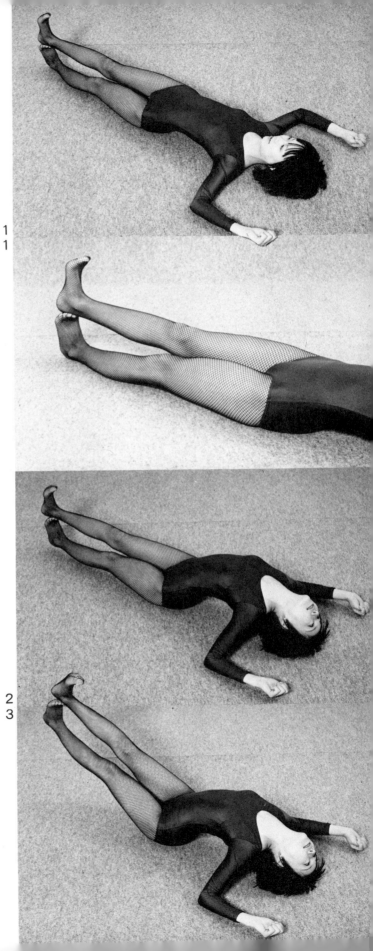

Movements and Breathing Order

1. Lying on your back, bend your right leg back till your right foot is close to your hips. Extend the Achilles' tendons of both feet. Your left foot is held straight. Grip your right ankle with your right hand and put your left hand on your abdomen.

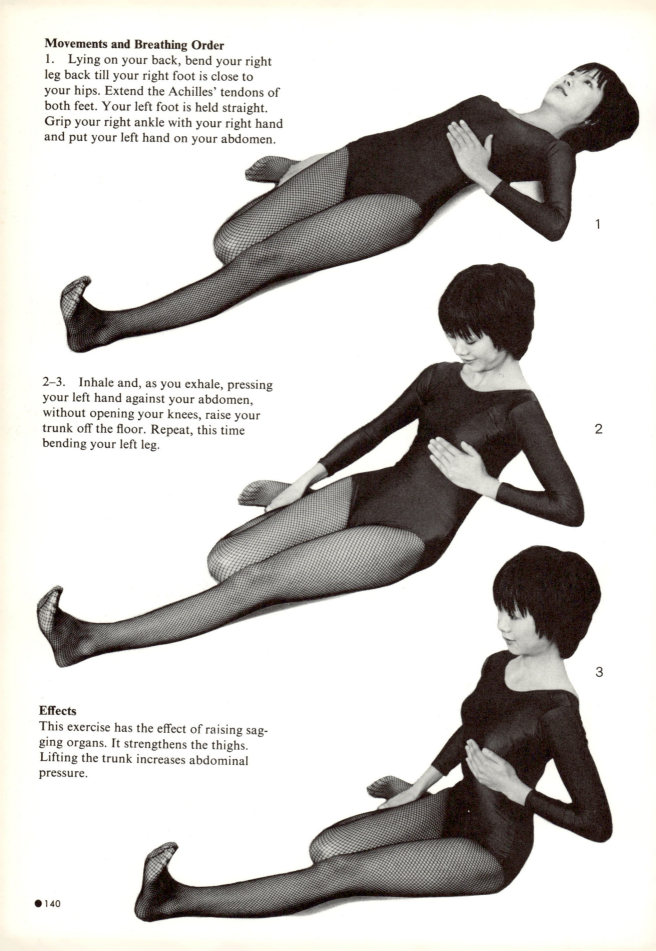

1

2–3. Inhale and, as you exhale, pressing your left hand against your abdomen, without opening your knees, raise your trunk off the floor. Repeat, this time bending your left leg.

2

3

Effects

This exercise has the effect of raising sagging organs. It strengthens the thighs. Lifting the trunk increases abdominal pressure.

Movements and Breathing Order

1. Lying on your back, hug your knees to your chest and regulate your breathing.

2. Inhale and, as you exhale, lift your head. At the same time, pull your legs with both arms to bring chin and knees together.

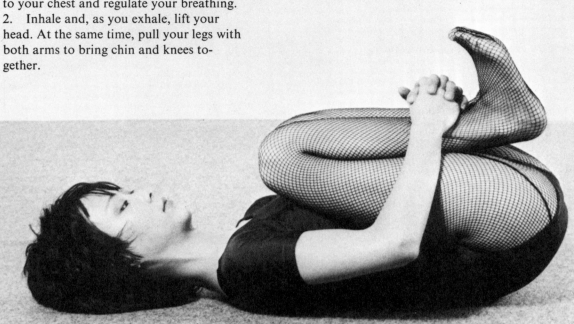

1

2

Effects

Stimulating the stomach and increasing abdominal pressure, this exercise limbers the back.

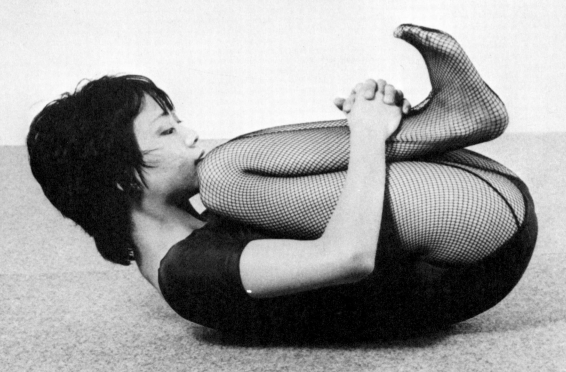

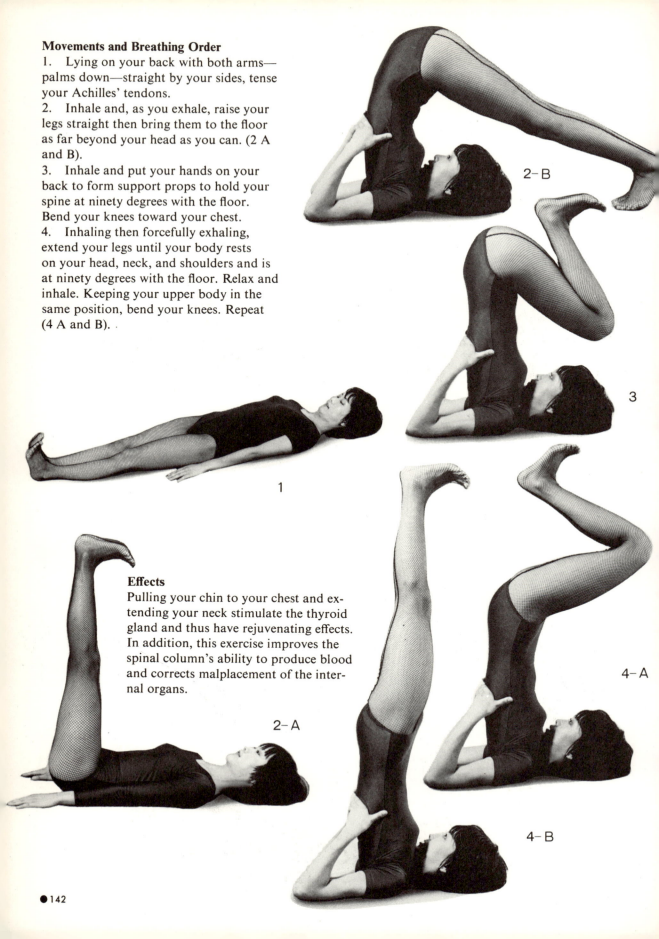

Movements and Breathing Order

1. Lying on your back with both arms—palms down—straight by your sides, tense your Achilles' tendons.
2. Inhale and, as you exhale, raise your legs straight then bring them to the floor as far beyond your head as you can. (2 A and B).
3. Inhale and put your hands on your back to form support props to hold your spine at ninety degrees with the floor. Bend your knees toward your chest.
4. Inhaling then forcefully exhaling, extend your legs until your body rests on your head, neck, and shoulders and is at ninety degrees with the floor. Relax and inhale. Keeping your upper body in the same position, bend your knees. Repeat (4 A and B).

Effects

Pulling your chin to your chest and extending your neck stimulate the thyroid gland and thus have rejuvenating effects. In addition, this exercise improves the spinal column's ability to produce blood and corrects malplacement of the internal organs.

2–B

3

1

2–A

4–A

4–B

Movements and Breathing Order

1. Lying on your stomach, bend your arms, elbows on the floor and both hands—palms down—under your chin. As you exhale, extend your knees and raise them about five centimeters off the floor.

2. Without raising your elbows from the floor, inhale then forcefully exhale as you extend your right leg. Raise it still further. Inhaling, return to the position in step 1.

3. Then, extending your left leg, raise it still further as you exhale. Repeat these movements several times.

Effects

This exercise increases abdominal pressure and strengthens the spinal column. In addition, it invigorates the endocrine system.

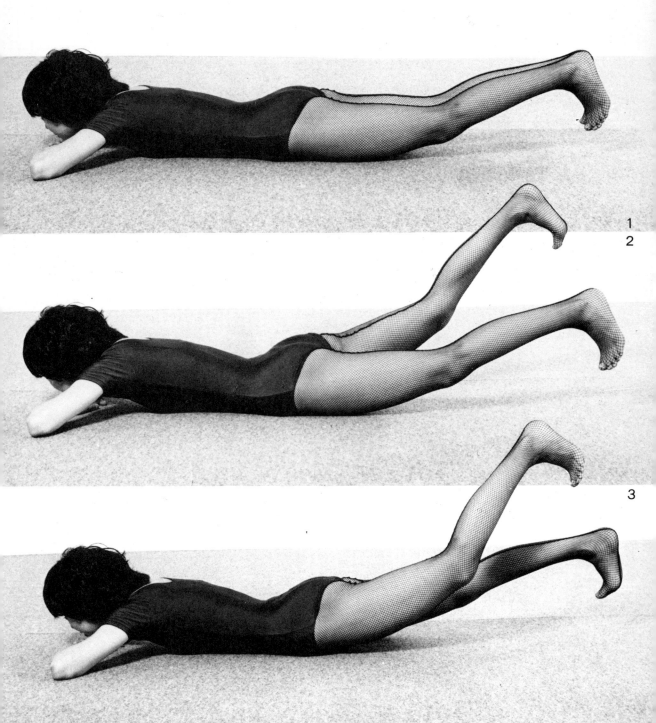

Movements and Breathing Order

1. Lying on your stomach with legs straight and together and Achilles' tendons tensed, join your hands in the prayer attitude behind your back. Put your forehead on the floor and regulate your breathing.

2. Exhaling, bend your upper body upward and backward. Thrusting your chest out, extend your neck fully forward. Allow your legs to open naturally. Do not bend your elbows at this time.

3–4. Inhale and, as you exhale, swing your legs to the right and left. Exhale as you swing them and inhale as you return them to the central position.

Effects

This exercise relieves blood congestion in the lower regions of the shoulder blades. Raising your legs prevents sagging of the interior organs. The right-left swing stimulates intestinal peristalsis.

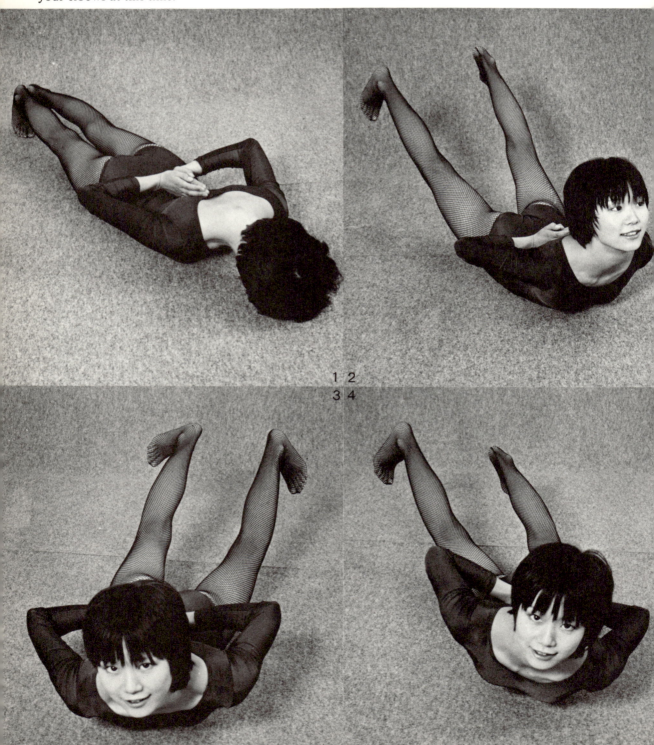

1 2
3 4

Movements and Breathing Order

1. Lying on your stomach, bend your right leg and bring the sole of your right foot to your left knee. Join your hands in the prayer attitude behind your back and put your forehead on the floor as you inhale.

2. Exhaling, raise your trunk and your left leg. Do not allow your right knee to leave the floor at this time. When you have completely exhaled, relax and return to the position in step 1.

3–4. Repeat, bending the left leg.

Effects

This exercise strengthens the side opposite the one on which the leg is raised. Further it relieves blood congestion on the same side and prevents sagging of the internal organs. It stimulates the cervical region and relieves stiffness in the neck and shoulders.

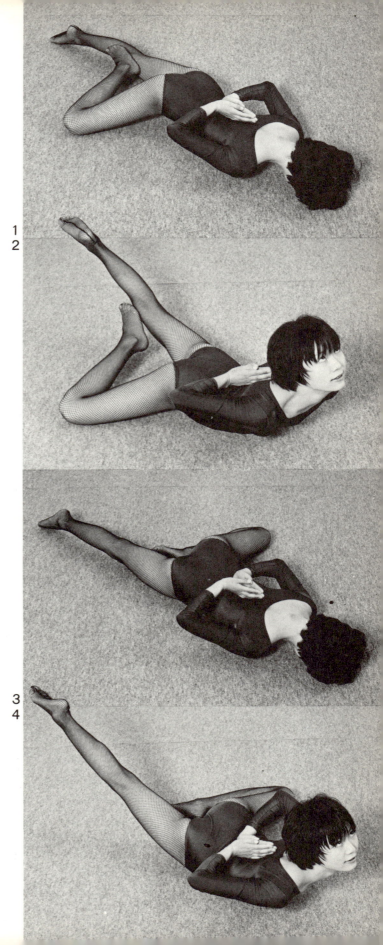

1
2

3
4

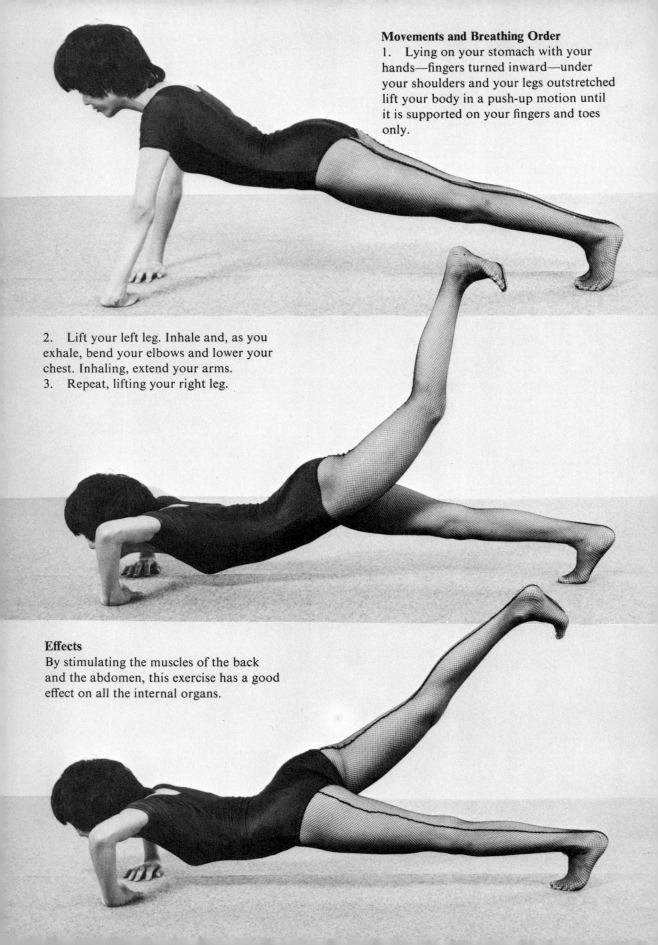

Movements and Breathing Order

1. Lying on your stomach with your hands—fingers turned inward—under your shoulders and your legs outstretched lift your body in a push-up motion until it is supported on your fingers and toes only.

2. Lift your left leg. Inhale and, as you exhale, bend your elbows and lower your chest. Inhaling, extend your arms.
3. Repeat, lifting your right leg.

Effects

By stimulating the muscles of the back and the abdomen, this exercise has a good effect on all the internal organs.

Movements and Breathing Order

1. Kneeling with your upper body and thighs straight and your feet spread behind you, put your hands on the lower border of your rib cage.

2. Exhaling, bend over backward as if you were pushing on your ribs. Your feet remain in the same position.

3. When you have leaned as far as possible, inhale. Then, exhaling again. swing your upper body to the right and left. At this time, you must keep your elbows as close to your body as possible and fully open your rib cage.

Effects

This exercise relieves contraction in the chest. Since it tenses the hip region, it stimulates the sacral vertebrae, improves the functioning of the reproductive system, and relieves blood congestion in the back.

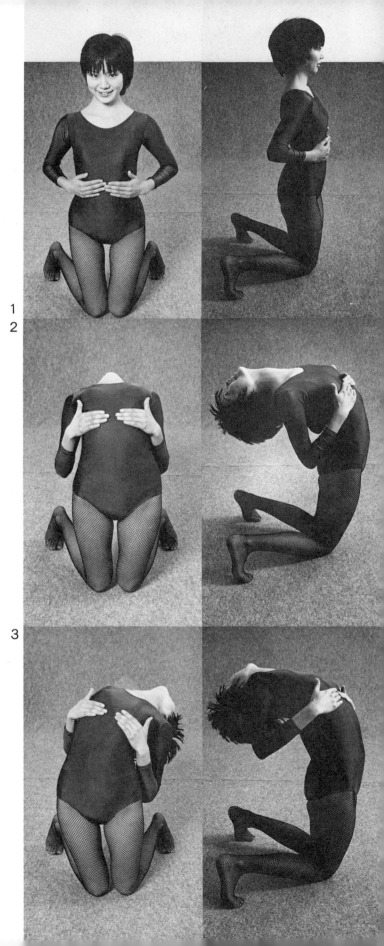

1
2

3

Pain in the Hips and Back

Goals and Effects

Pain in the back and hips are not only among the most frequent, but also among the hardest to understand and the most difficult to cure. Among older people, slipped vertebrae, muscular ailments, and irregularities in internal organs are frequent causes; but the trouble may be any of about two hundred other things ranging from flat feet to cancer. Of course, treatment differs according to the cause; but, in general, the following kinds of exercises are employed: movements centering on the hips and backs in order to strengthen the muscles and correct posture; motions to limber stiff muscles; and breathing exercises to increase abdominal pressure, improve circulation of the blood, and strengthen muscles. Special attention is devoted to curing constipation and sagging of the internal organs. It is important to avoid excessively acid foods and to ensure that the body gets sufficient calcium.

Movements and Breathing Order

1. Kneeling in the *seiza* position with your head forward, stretch your back, pull in your chin, and join your hands high over your head.
2. Inhale and, as you exhale, lean your upper body to the right so as to lower your left hip. Stretch well until your hands form a straight line. At this time, keep your upper arms in line with your ears.
3. Inhaling, return your trunk to the vertical positon. Then, exhaling, bend your upper body to the left so as to lower your right hip.

Effects

Bending your body to the side, limbers your backbone, improves circulation, and corrects spinal inclination to the right or left.

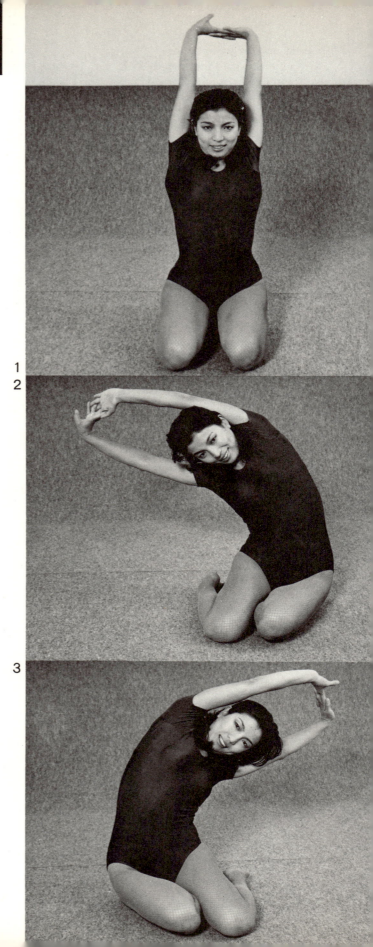

1
2
3

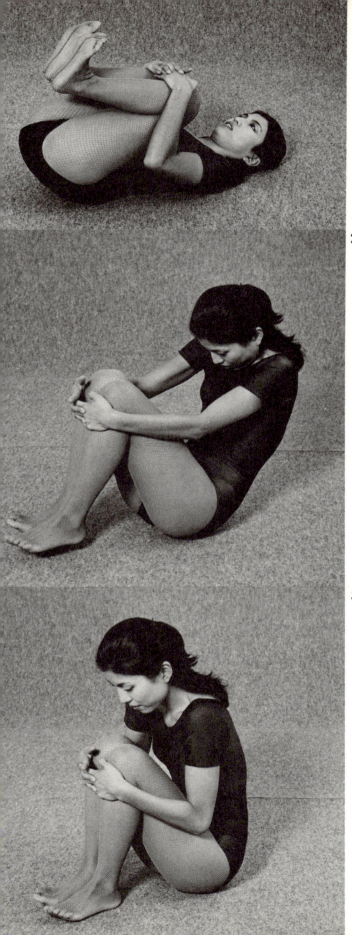

1
2

3

Movements and Breathing Order

1.   Lying on your back, extend your Achilles' tendons and, wrapping your arms around them, pull your knees toward your chest.

2–3.   Inhale and, as you exhale, still embracing your knees, raise your upper body. Inhale and, as you exhale, return to the position in step 1. Repeat several times.

Effects

This exercise limbers the spinal column, massages the back muscles, improves circulation, and relieves stiffness in the back.

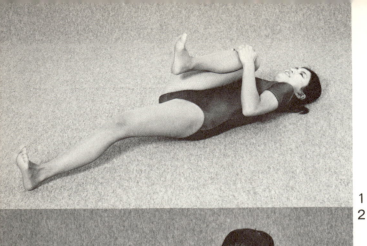

1
2

Movements and Breathing Order

1. Lying on your back, extend your Achilles' tendons and pull your right knee toward your chest.

2. Inhale and, as you exhale, still embracing your right knee, raise your upper body.

3–4. Returning to the position in step 1, next pull your left knee toward your chest and repeat.

Effects

This exercise cures irregularities in blood circulation and relieves hip and back pain caused by abnormalities in the abdomen.

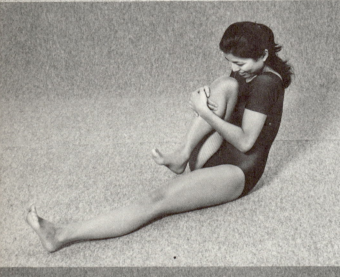

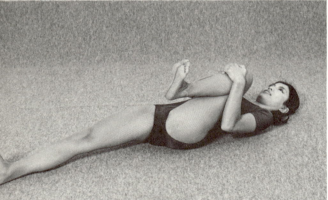

3
4

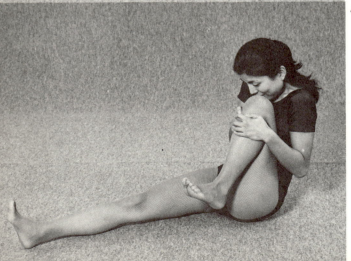

Movements and Breathing Order

1. Lying on your back, put your right hand behind your neck and put your right foot on top of your left knee. Put your left hand on your right knee.

2. Inhale and, as you exhale, touch the floor on the left side with your right knee; turn your face to the right. Do not allow your right elbow to leave the floor. Inhaling, return your right knee to the position in step 1.

3–4. Repeat with the left knee.

Effects

This exercise cures organic displacement caused by twists in the hip region and relieves stress brought on by this irregularity.

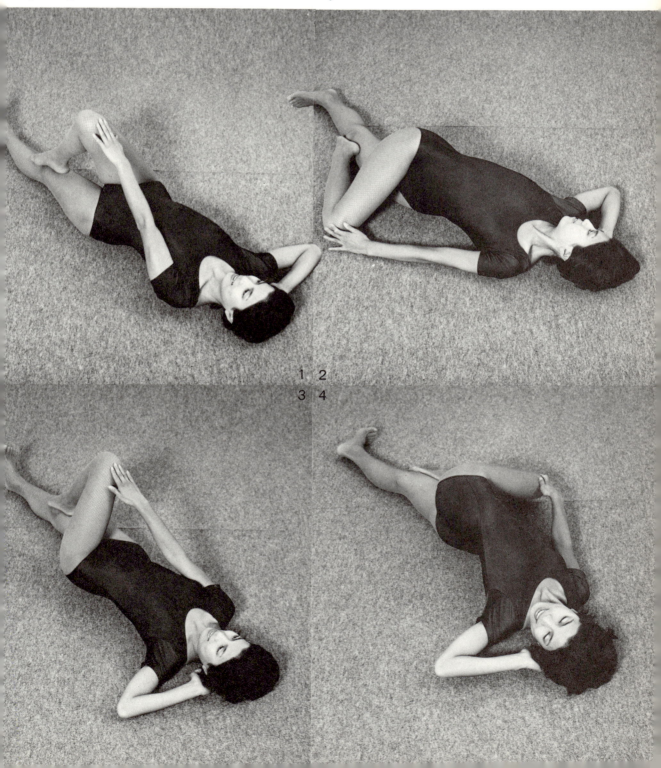

1 2
3 4

Movements and Breathing Order

1. Lying on your back with your legs together, fully extend your Achilles' tendons and join your hand behind your neck so that both elbows lie on the floor.
2. Inhale and, as you exhale, without bending the knee, raise your right leg until it is perpendicular to the floor.
3. Inhale and, as you exhale, swing your right foot to the floor on your left side. At the same time, turn your face to the right.

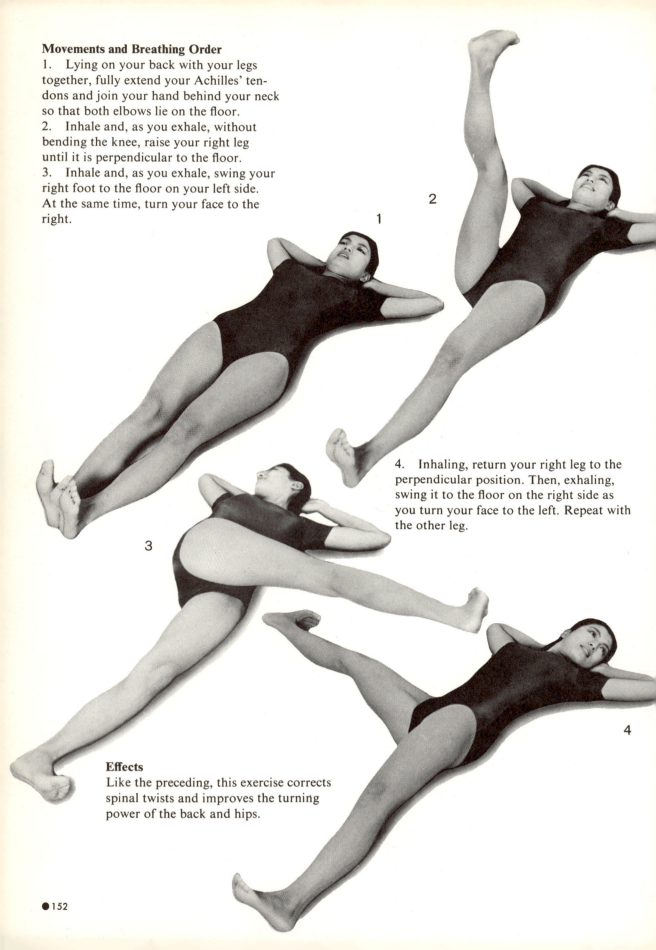

4. Inhaling, return your right leg to the perpendicular position. Then, exhaling, swing it to the floor on the right side as you turn your face to the left. Repeat with the other leg.

Effects

Like the preceding, this exercise corrects spinal twists and improves the turning power of the back and hips.

Movements and Breathing Order

1.   Lying on your back with both legs together and your Achilles' tendons extended, join your hand behind your neck and extend your elbows to your sides.

2.   Inhale and, as you exhale, raise your hips so that your body is supported on your heels and elbows.

3.   Inhale and, as you exhale, twist your hips to the left and turn your face to the right.

4.   Inhaling, return your body to the position in step 2. Then, as you exhale, twist your hips to the right and turn your face to the left.

5.   Gradually spread your feet as you repeat this exercise.

Effects

This exercise limbers the back and hips and corrects twists. By spreading your feet gradually, you cause stimulation to move from the upper part of the spine downward.

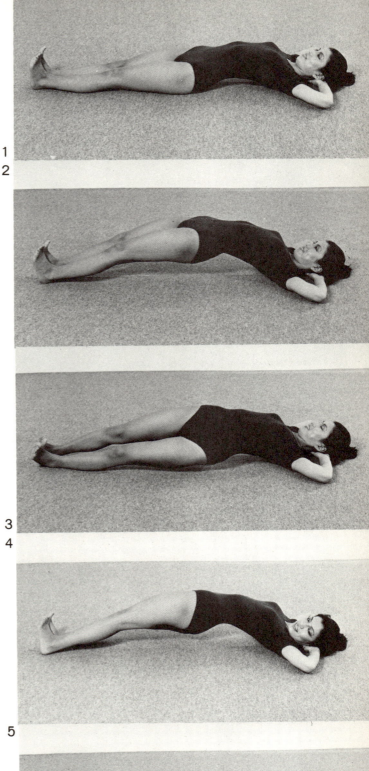

1
2
3
4
5

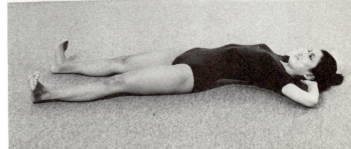

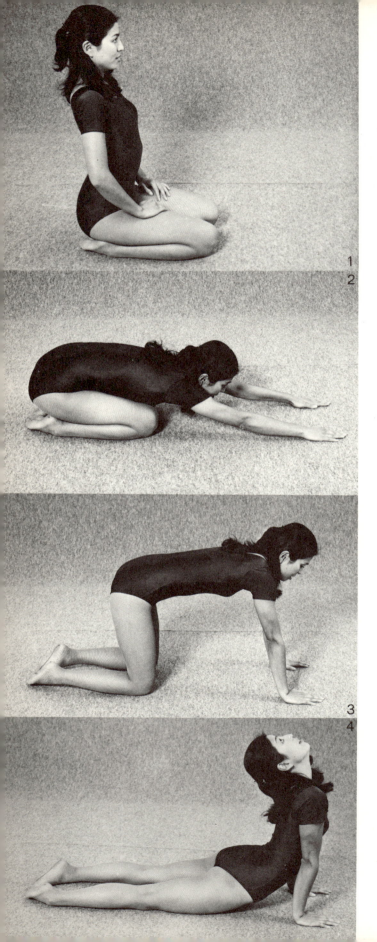

Movements and Breathing Order

1. Kneeling in the *seiza* position with neck and back held straight and with chest thrust forward, pull your chin inward, look to the front, and regulate your breathing. Put your hands on your knees or thighs.
2. Inhale and, as you exhale, slide both hands to the floor in front of you and extend your upper body well to the front.
3–4. Inhale and, as you exhale, crouch on all fours. From this posture, thrusting your chin forward, lower your hips to the floor and bend your trunk backward. Inhaling and without changing your hand position, raise your hips till you are once again crouching on all fours. Then lower your hips to the rear to return your body to the position in step 2. Inhale fully as you keep your arms extended. During this reversal of steps 2 through 4, breathe rhythmically.

Effects

Since, like the cat posture, this exercise causes a wave motion along the entire spinal column and moves the back forward and rearward, it limbers both hips and spine.

Movements and Breathing Order ▶

1. Lying on your stomach with legs together and Achilles' tendons extended, put your hands by your sides under your shoulders and bring your elbows close to your body. Put your forehead on the floor.
2. Inhaling, thrust your chin forward. As you bend your back upward and to the rear, raise both legs without allowing your knees to leave the floor.
3. Exhaling and remaining in the same position, raise your right leg still further upward and to the side. Inhaling, return your right leg to the position in step 2.
4. As you exhale, repeat with your left leg. Execute steps 3 through 4 with your upper body bent as far upward and to the rear as possible.

Effects

This variation of the cobra pose stimulates the hips and back. Gradually spreading one leg to the side changes the location of stimulation and concentrates it on the side toward which the leg moves.

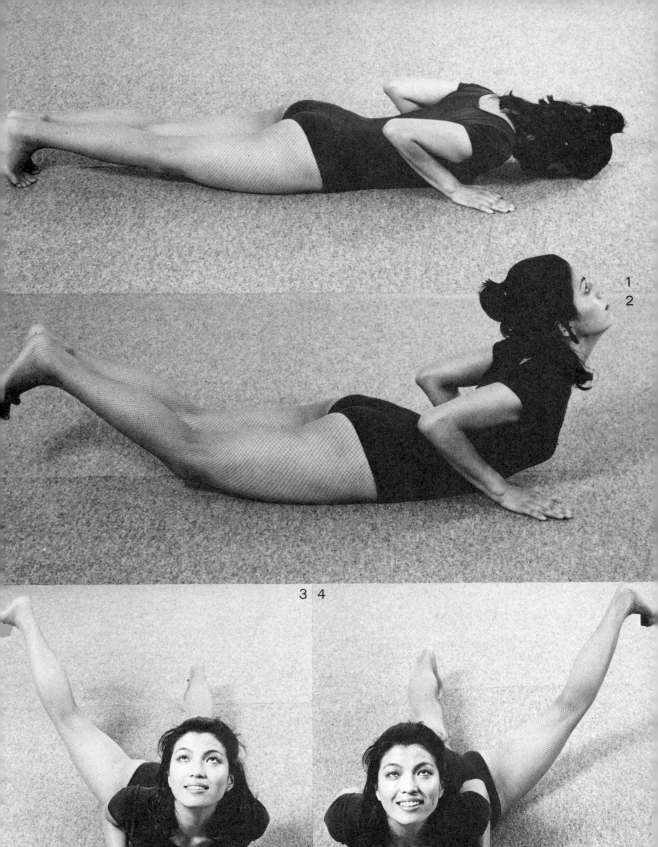

1
2

3 4

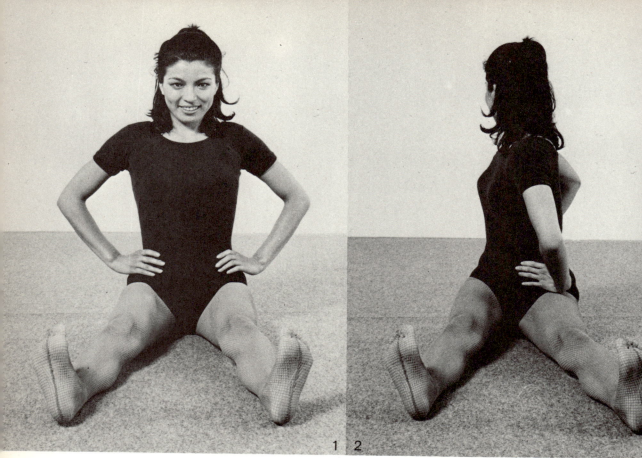

1 2

Movements and Breathing Order

1. Sitting straight up with both legs extended and spread in front of you, put both hands behind your neck, extend your elbows to the sides, and lean forward.
2. Inhale and, as you exhale, twist your upper body to the right until your elbows form a line perpendicular with the floor. Your face must be turned straight to the side.
3. Inhale and return your body to the position in step 1. Inhale and, as you exhale, twist your body to the left in the same fashion.

Effects

This exercise limbers the back and corrects twists. It stimulates the upper part of the back.

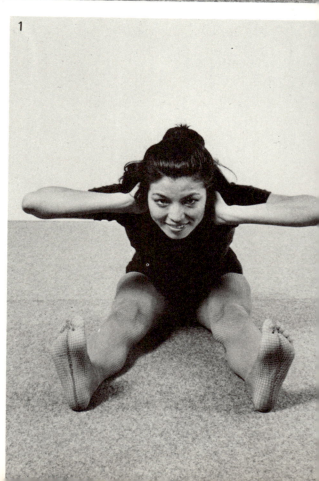

1

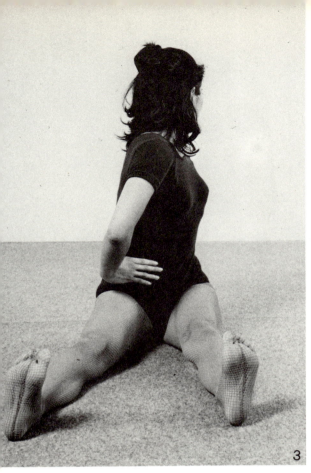

Movements and Breathing Order

1. Sitting on the floor with both legs extended in front of you and spread to about the width of your hips, put your hands on your hips, look straight forward, and regulate your breathing.
2. Inhale and, as you exhale, turn your body to the right from your hips. Look to the rear.
3. Inhaling, return your body to the position in step 1. Inhale and, as you exhale, twist your body to the left in the same fashion.

Effects

Twisting your hips and back in this way limbers this part of your body and corrects irregularities. Spreading your legs lowers the point of stimulation.

3

2 3

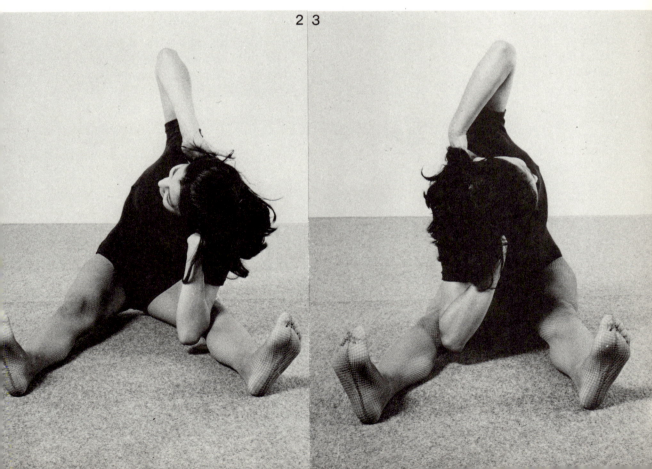

Movements and Breathing Order

1. Sitting straight with both legs spread wide, extend the Achilles' tendon of your right foot and bend your left leg inward so that the left foot comes to the center of your body. Holding neck and back straight, pull your chin in, look straight forward, and regulate your breathing.

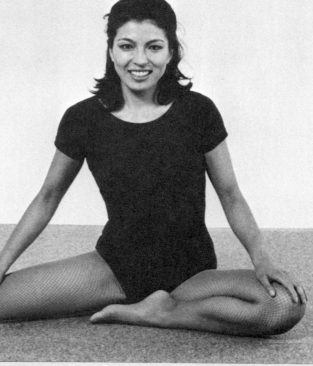

1

2

2. Turn your upper body to the right. Then, gripping the heel of your right foot with both hands, bend over to the right as you inhale and then exhale. Without bending your right knee, try to bring your forehead and chest to your right leg. Inhaling, return your upper body to the vertical position, outstretch your left leg, bend your right leg inward, and repeat to the left side.

Effects

While extending and limbering the back and hips, this exercise corrects right and left deviation of the internal organs, regulates the ability of the pelvis to open and close, and relieves contraction in the muscles of the undersides of the feet.

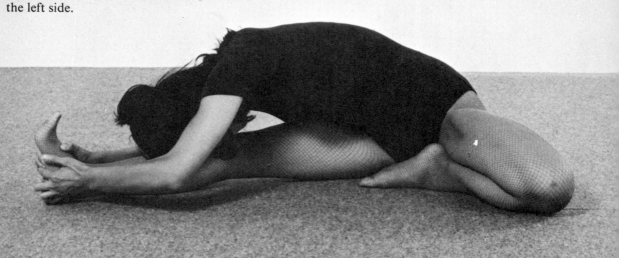

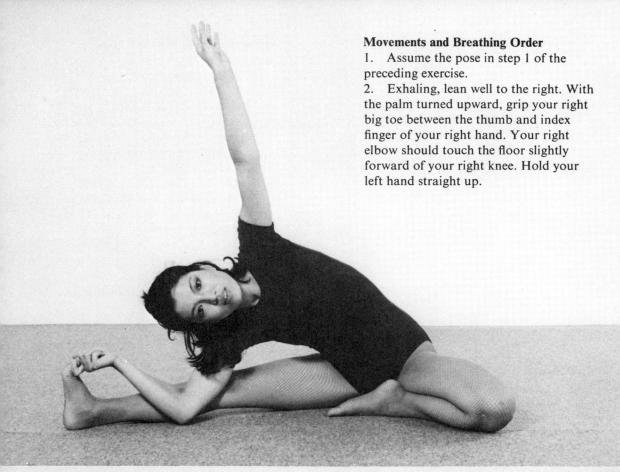

Movements and Breathing Order

1. Assume the pose in step 1 of the preceding exercise.

2. Exhaling, lean well to the right. With the palm turned upward, grip your right big toe between the thumb and index finger of your right hand. Your right elbow should touch the floor slightly forward of your right knee. Hold your left hand straight up.

3. Inhale and, as you exhale, lower your left hand to the right until you bring it to your right hand. Your left arm must be in line with your left ear. Fully stretch your left side. Inhaling, return to the position in step 1 and repeat to the other side.

Effects

By extending the sides of the abdomen and regulating the ribs, this exercise relieves strain in the hips and back.

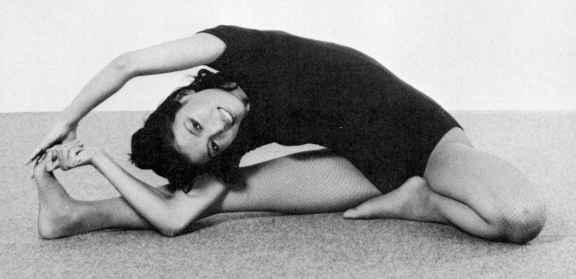

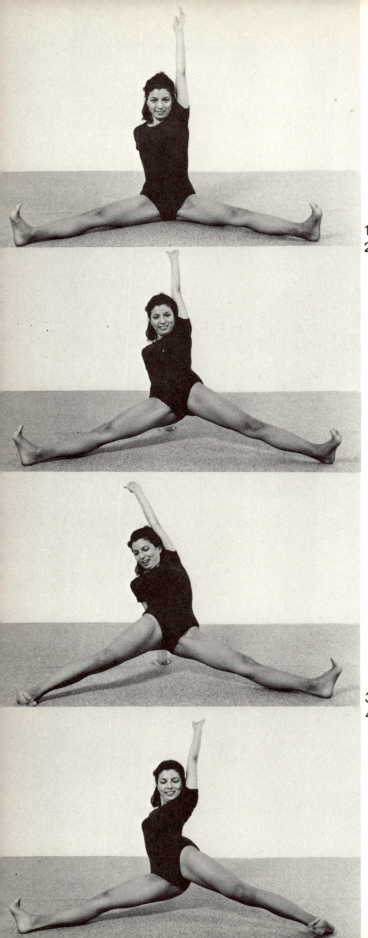

Movements and Breathing Order

1. Sitting straight with your legs spread wide in front of you, raise your left hand straight up and put your right hand on the floor behind you.

2. Inhale and, as you exhale, raise your hips from the floor and thrust your abdomen and chest forward. Bringing your left arm to your left ear, lean slightly rearward, keep your face forward, and pull your chin in.

3. Inhale and, as you exhale, twist your hips to the left. Inhaling, return to the position in step 2.

4. Exhaling, twist your hips to the right. Repeat, raising your right hand and putting your left hand on the floor behind you.

Effects

By raising your hips with your legs spread wide, this exercise strengthens the hip region. The twisting motion improves hip flexibility. Circulation is improved on the side on which the arm is raised.

Movements and Breathing Order ▶

1. Kneel on all fours with knees together and with hands pointed straight forward.

2–3. Inhale and, as you exhale, raise your right hand and right leg as high as you can. Then swing your right leg to the left as if you were going to put it on the floor. Exhale fully. Inhaling, return your body to the position in step 2. Then return to the position in step 1. Repeat the exercise, raising the left arm and leg.

Effects

The side of the back on which the leg and arm are outstretched and the opposite hip are stimulated. This exercise firms the muscles of the hips and back and improves their balance.

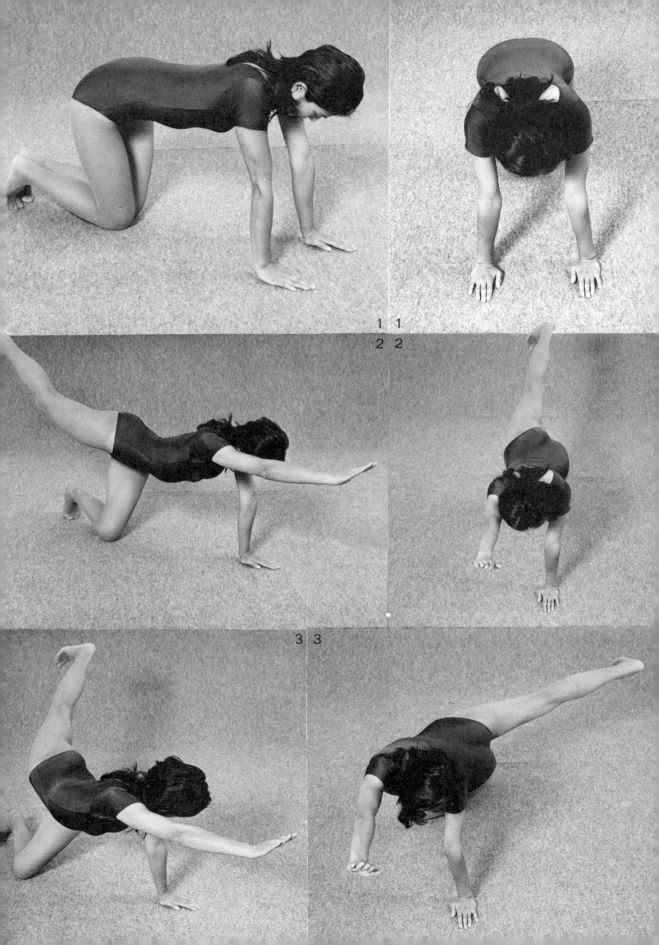

1 1
2 2

3 3

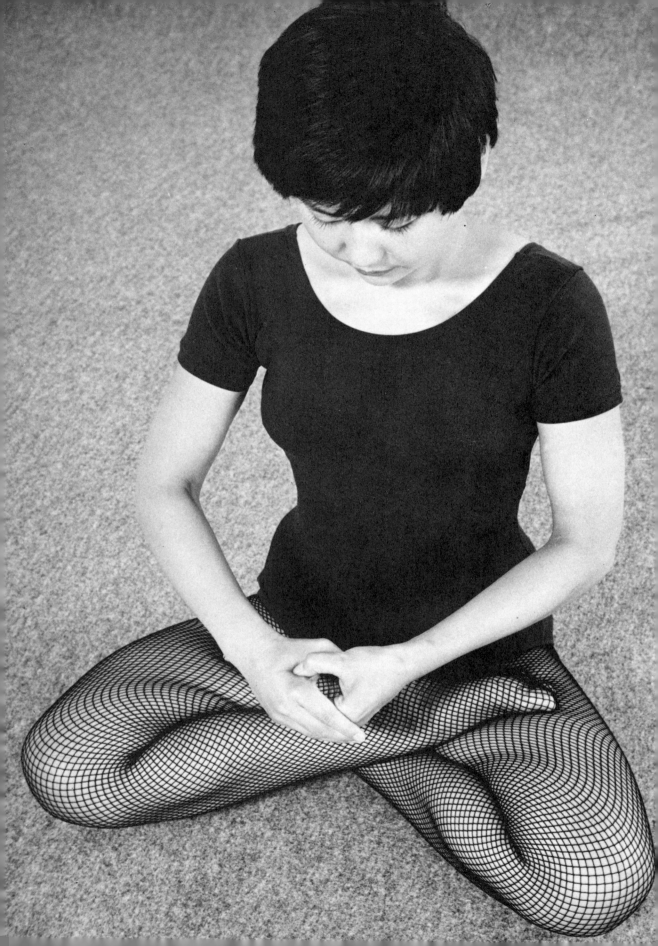

Constipation

Goals and Effects

Constipation, which can set up a viscious circle of other pathological reactions, arises from ailments of the intestines or from irregularities in such other organs as the liver and the stomach. As the tradition to the effect that constipation is the source of all other illnesses suggests, causes and treatment must be sought in and applied to the entire body. But the exercises below treat constipation caused by slackness, contraction, debility, displacement, or adhesions of the intestines. In addition to curing these conditions, they increase abdominal pressure, improve circulation in the hips and abdomen, and activate the nervous and endocrine systems. Strengthening the hips improves the functioning of the internal organs, activates intestinal peristalsis and the operation of the kidneys, and thus improves evacuation.

◀ Movements and Breathing Order

Sit in the cross-legged position used in Zen meditation. Relaxing your shoulders and neck, regulate your breathing. Tense the inner sides of your thighs. Have the feeling that you are lifting something with your knees and concentrate strength in your diaphragm. With your left thumb, rub and press the fork between your right thumb and index finger. Then rub the fork between your left thumb and index finger.

Effects

This exercise promotes mental stability. Rubbing the fork between the thumb and index finger stimulates the large intestine and thus helps bring about evacuation.

▲ Movements and Breathing Order

Sitting in the cross-legged position used in Zen meditation, clench your fists, thumbs inside. Lightly tap the top of your head with your right fist (do not strike your head hard). Exhale as you tap. Repeat with the left fist.

Effects

Tapping on the head stimulates the intestines and helps bring about evacuation.

Movements and Breathing Order

1. Sitting in the cross-legged position used in Zen meditation, put your hands on the floor beside your thighs.
2. Pulling your chin in and supporting yourself only on your hands, lift your body. Concentrate strength in your diaphragm, do *kumbhaka*, or retain the breath, and hold the pose as long as you can. Then relax.

Effects

This exercise has the effect of correcting sagging of the rib cage and the internal organs. *Kumbhaka* increases abdominal pressure.

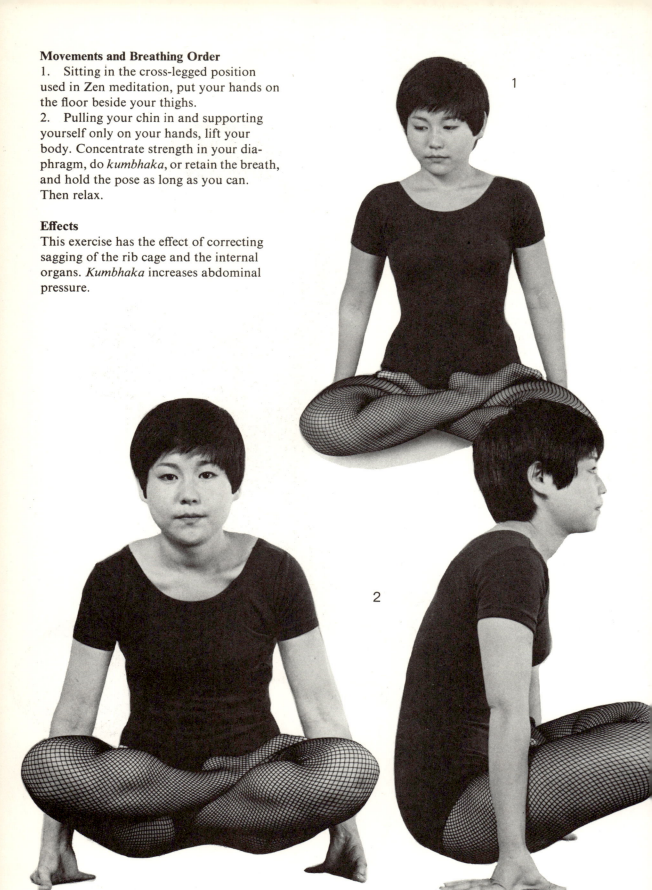

Movements and Breathing Order

With your hands on your hips, stand straight with feet together. Then jump upward. At the same time, tap your hips with your heels. Exhaling strongly, repeat.

Effects

This movement stimulates the kidneys and improves the functioning of the intestines by stimulating peristalsis.

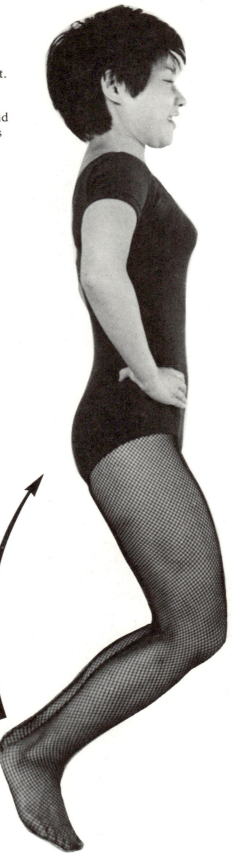

Movements and Breathing Order

1. Stand with both feet spread wide and with hands joined—palms upward—over your head. Inhale deep.

2–3. Exhaling, keeping your chin pointed forward and without bending your knees, lean diagonally forward as far as possible, then swing your body to the right.

4–7. With arms fully extended and upper body straight, swing your trunk upward till your arms are straight above you. Lean as far to the rear as possible.

8–11. Exhaling, swing your body in the opposite direction until it is in the position in step 2. Concentrate on your pelvis throughout these motions.

Effects

Fatigue and aging cause the muscles of the undersides of the feet to contract. This exercise relieves this condition and, by improving the right-left opening ability of the pelvis, stimulates the intestines.

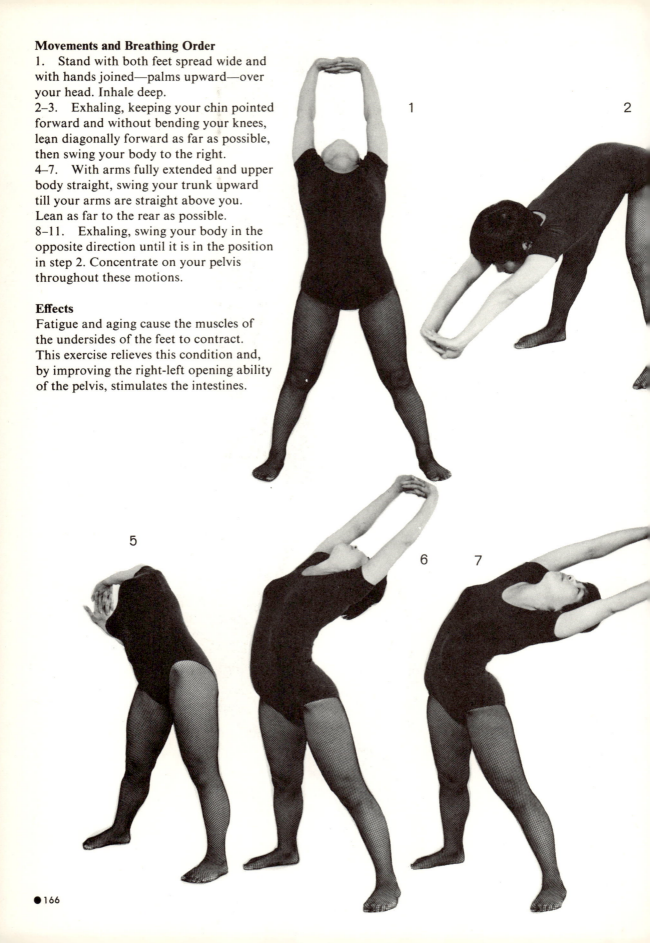

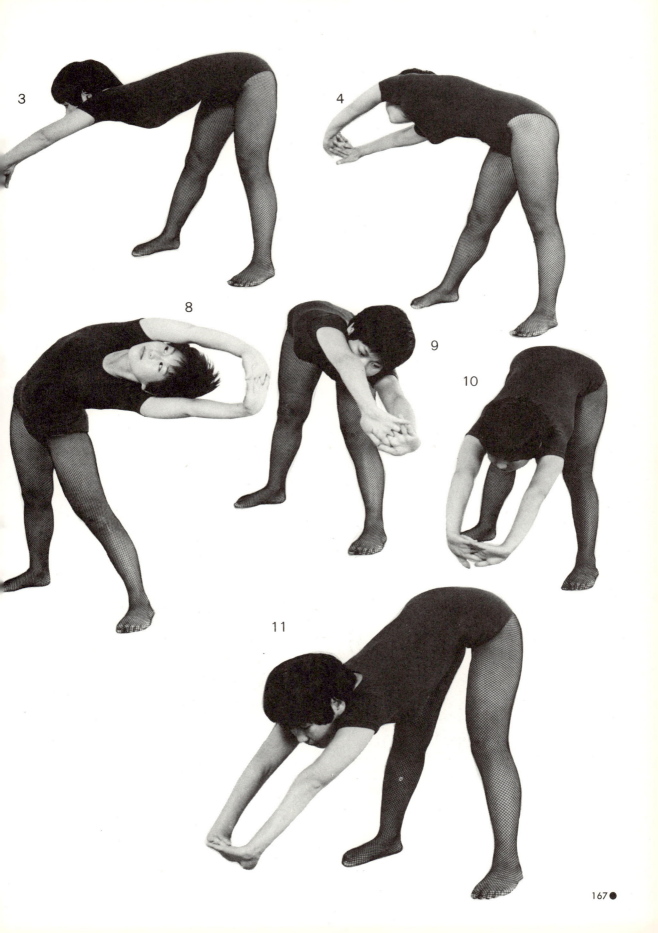

3

4

8

9

10

11

Movements and Breathing Order

Kneel with your buttocks between your feet and then lean over till your trunk and face are turned upward. Put your clenched right fist on your abdomen. Stretch your left arm out on the floor above your head. Raise your hips, inhale deeply, and do *kumbhaka*. Deliberately concentrating on your right abdomen, tap it with your right fist. At the same time, exhale forcefully and extend your left arm still further upward. Repeat, extending your right arm above your head and tapping your abdomen with your left fist.

Effects

This exercise relieves congestion of blood in the abdomen. Tapping strengthens the muscles and improves evacuation.

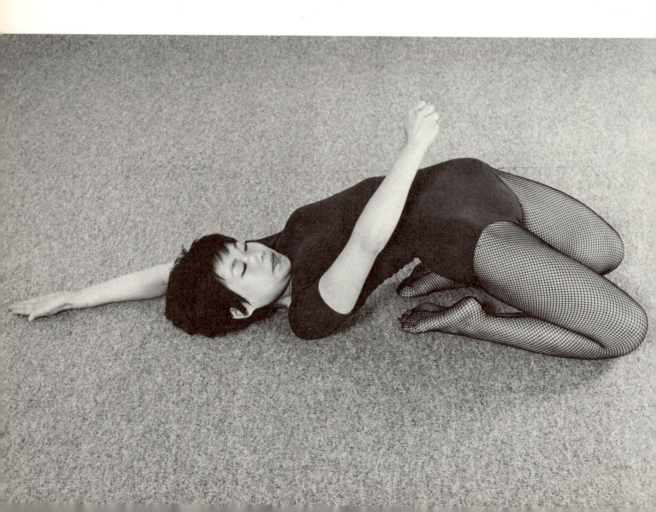

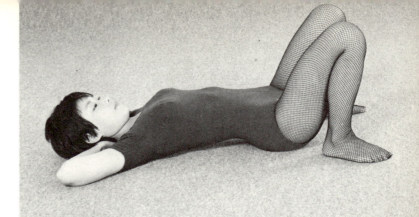

1

2

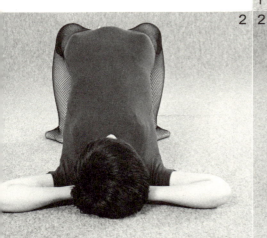

2

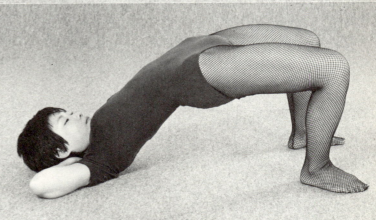

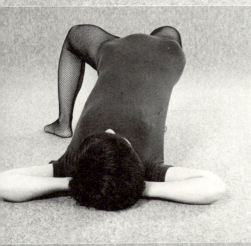

3-A
3-B

Movements and Breathing Order

1. Lying on your back with your knees raised, join both hands behind your neck.
2. Inhaling deeply, raise your hips and abdomen. With your heels on the floor, do *kumbhaka* and deliberately concentrate on your diaphragm.
3. Forcefully exhale and, without relaxing your diaphragm, deliberately concentrate on your pelvis. Swing your hips to one side then lower them (3 A and B). Do not allow your elbows or shoulders to leave the floor. Repeat, swinging your hips in the opposite direction.

Effects

Strengthening muscles and improving the functioning of the internal organs, this exercise corrects sagging, increases abdominal pressure, and relieves constipation.

Movements and Breathing Order

1. Lying on your back and extending both Achilles' tendons, pull your right knee toward your chest with both hands. Inhale deeply.

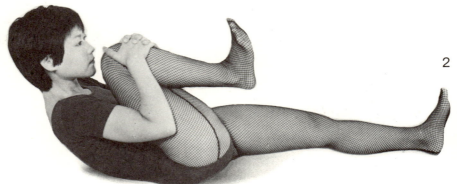

1

2

2–3. Exhaling forcefully and still pulling your knee to your chest, sit up. At this time, fully extend the Achilles' tendon and muscles of the underside of your left foot. Repeat, pulling your left knee to your chest and keeping your right leg straight.

Effects

This exercise strengthens the abdomen, relieves blood congestion, passes gas, and stimulates intestinal peristalsis.

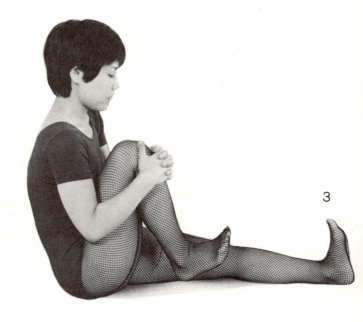

3

Movements and Breathing Order

1. Lying on your back, tuck your chin in, join both hands behind your neck, and with both legs together and straight extend your Achilles' tendons.

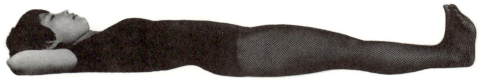

2. Inhaling deeply, fully extend the Achilles' tendons of both feet. Raise your feet off the floor to the height shown in the photography. Do *Kumbhaka* and concentrate awareness in your diaphragm.

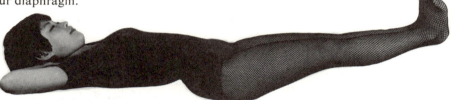

3–4. Without relaxing your diaphragm, exhale strongly as you raise and lower your feet, gradually spreading your legs farther apart. Do not let your elbows or shoulders leave the floor. When your legs are spread as far as possible, still raising and lowering them, gradually return them to the position in step 2. Repeat steps 2 through 4. When you have returned your legs to the position in step 2 for a second time, quietly lower them to the floor.

Effects

Tensing the abdomen and legs strengthens the muscles and the internal organs. The wider your legs are spread, the lower the stimulus this exercise provides. This encourages evacuation.

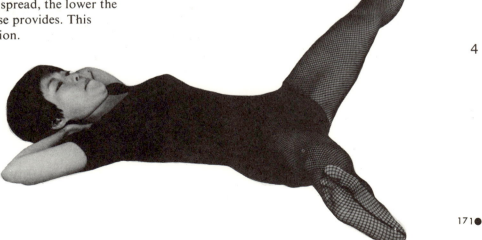

Movements and Breathing Order

1. Lying on your back, spread your arms, palms down, straight to the sides, as if they were supporting your body. Tensing your Achilles' tendons, raise both legs together till they are perpendicular to the floor. Inhaling deeply, do *kumbhaka* and concentrate strength in your diaphragm.

2. Without relaxing your diaphragm, exhale forcefully and concentrate deliberately on your hips. Holding them together lower both legs until they almost touch the floor on the right side. Turn your face to the left. Inhaling, return to the position in step 1. Do not allow your right shoulder to leave the floor when you lower your legs to the left and vice versa.

1

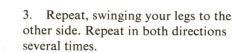

2

3. Repeat, swinging your legs to the other side. Repeat in both directions several times.

Effects

Swinging your legs to one side then the other stimulates and strengthens the muscles of the legs and feet and improves intestinal peristalsis.

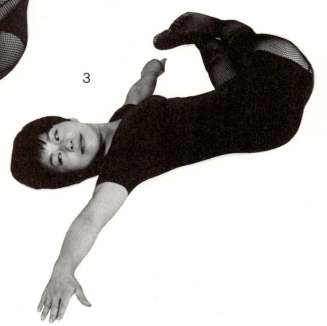

3

Movements and Breathing Order

1. Kneel on all fours with hands apart at about shoulder width and with knees together. Thrust your chest forward. With heels together, extend your Achilles' tendons and open your knees. Look forward and inhale.

2. As you exhale, lower your feet to the right. Twist your hips and head in the direction in which you lower your feet so that you see your feet across your shoulder. Your arms must remain straight. When you have completely exhaled, inhale and return legs and head to the position in step 1.

3. Repeat, lowering your legs and looking in the opposite direction.

Effects

Twisting the abdomen, hips and back stimulates blood circulation in the abdomen, relieves congestion and adhesion, and improves intestinal peristalsis.

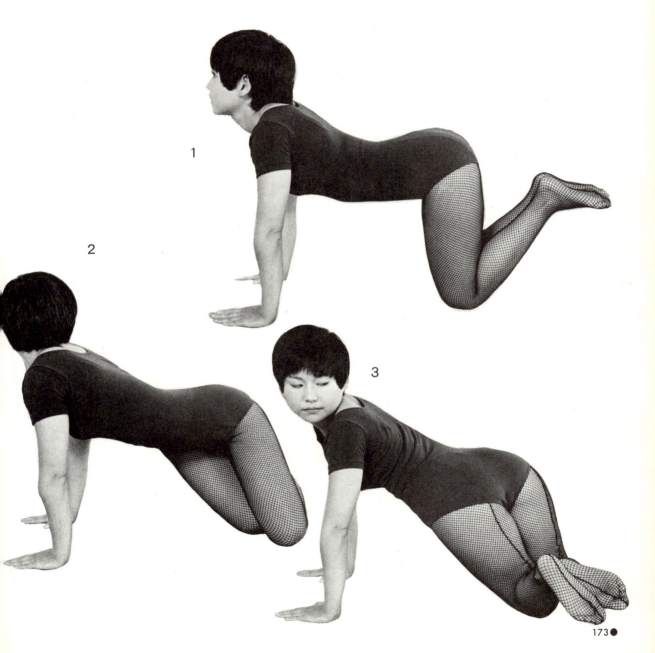

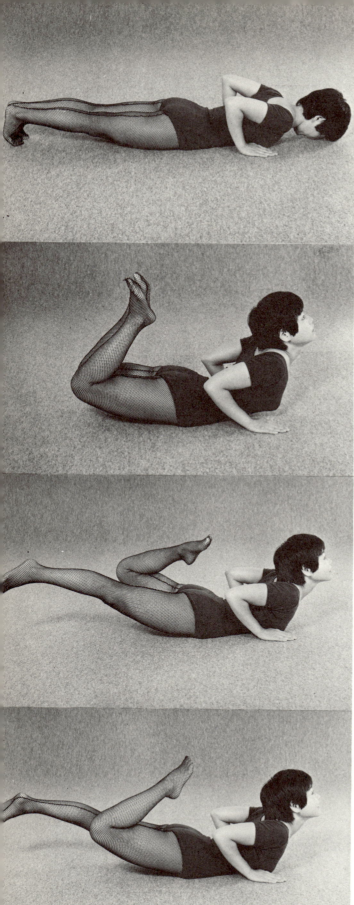

Movements and Breathing Order

1. Lying on your stomach with your head on the floor and your chin pulled in, put both hands on the floor beside your chest. Keep your elbows close to your sides.

2. Inhaling deeply, raise your upper body and your knees. Forcefully exhaling bend as if you were bringing your knees to your head.

3–4. When you have completely exhaled, bend first one leg then the other as if you were tapping your buttocks with your heels (3 A and B).

Effects

This exercise strengthens the abdominal muscles and relieves oppression in the internal organs and curvature of the lumbar vertebrae. It further stimulates circulation to the heart and improves both digestion and evacuation.

1
2

3–A

Movements and Breatning Order ▶

1. Standing with your legs spread as far as possible and your toes turned inward, lean forward and put your hands—fingers spread and pointed forward— on the floor well in front of you, your hands should be somewhat farther apart than your shoulders are wide. Extending your Achilles' tendons, without bending your knees, extend our elbows well. Inhaling, retract your buttocks. Extend the muscles of the undersides of your feet and bring your head between your arms. Pull your chin toward your chest.

2. Forecefully exhaling, straighten your elbows and your heels and lower your body almost to the floor. At the same time, bend your trunk and head backward. Thrust your chin forward. Repeat both steps 1 and 2.

Effects

Tensing and relaxing the hips stimulate and improve the functioning of the internal organs.

3–B

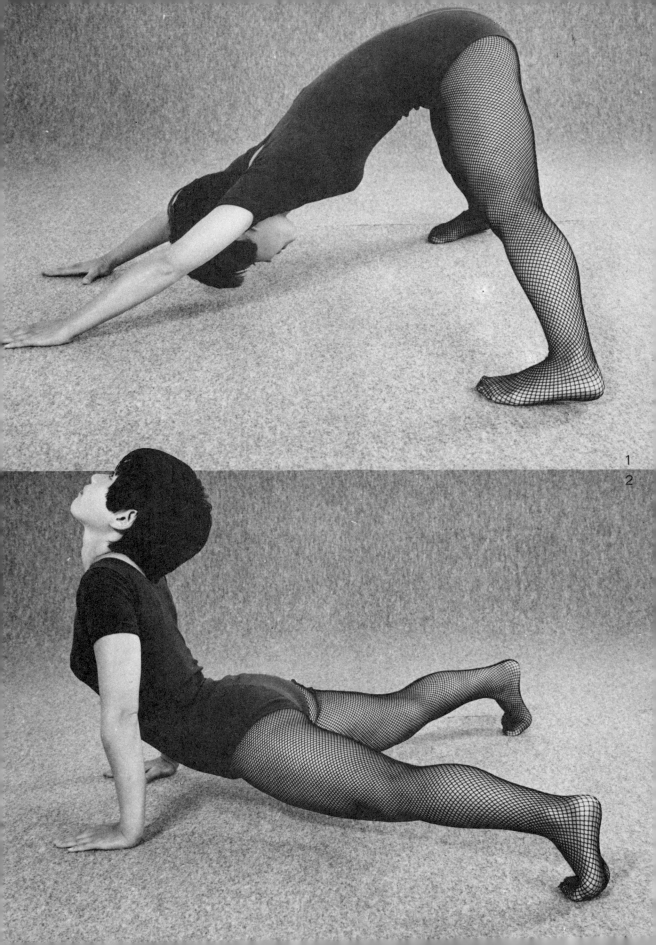

Movements and Breathing Order

1. Standing with your feet spread as wide as possible, with toes pointed inward, put your hands—fingers pointed forward—on the floor well in front of you. They should be somewhat farther apart than your shoulders are wide. Extend your elbows fully and, without bending your knees, extend your Achilles' tendons. As you inhale, retract your buttocks, extend the muscles of the undersides of your feet, and lower your head between your arms. Pull your chin toward your chest.

2. Holding your breath, without lowering your buttocks, bend your elbows. At the same time, lower your head till it almost touches the floor. Tense your big toes and the inner sides of your feet. Without lowering your hips, put your chin almost on the floor and thrust your body as far forward as possible.

3–4. As you exhale, suddenly drop your hips and straighten your elbows to bend you sharply upward and to the rear. Repeat.

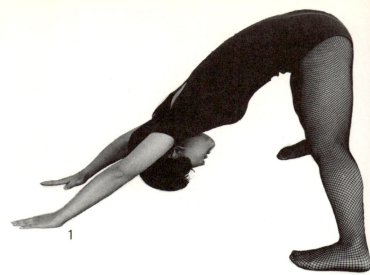

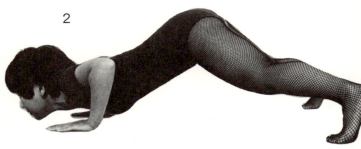

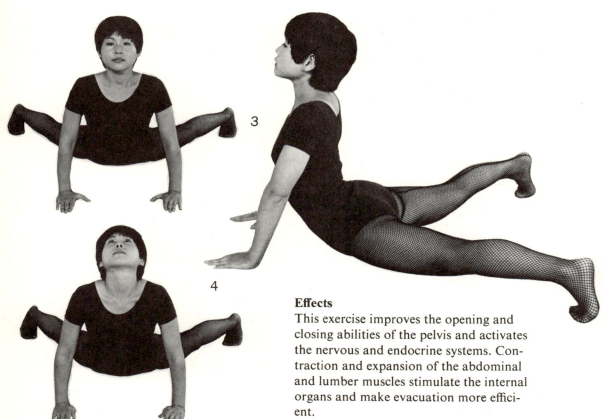

Effects

This exercise improves the opening and closing abilities of the pelvis and activates the nervous and endocrine systems. Contraction and expansion of the abdominal and lumber muscles stimulate the internal organs and make evacuation more efficient.

Movements and Breathing Order

1. Lying with legs spread wide and with toes on the floor, put your hands on the floor at about shoulder width and straighten your elbows. Keeping your arms perpendicular to the floor, lower your hips.

2. Exhaling, twist your upper body and head to the right and turn to look at your left heel. Lower both heels to the floor.

3. At the same time, twist your body in the opposite direction. Repeat these motions rapidly. Inhale when you return to the position in step 1.

Effects

Repeated strong twisting of the wrists, ankles, and hips activates the functioning of the intestines.

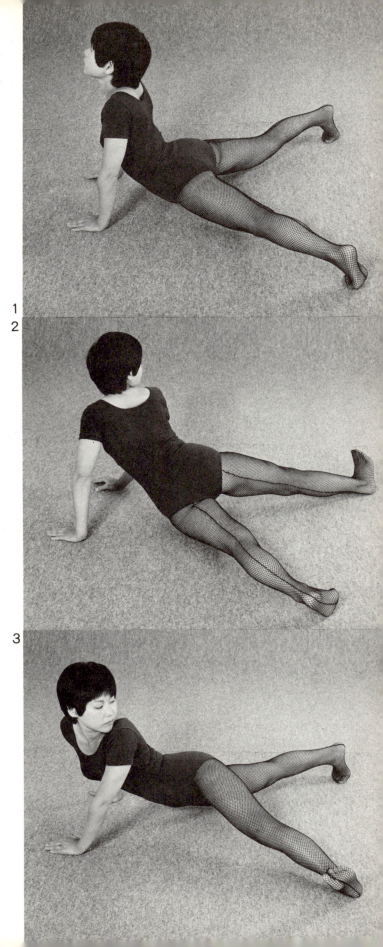

1

2

3

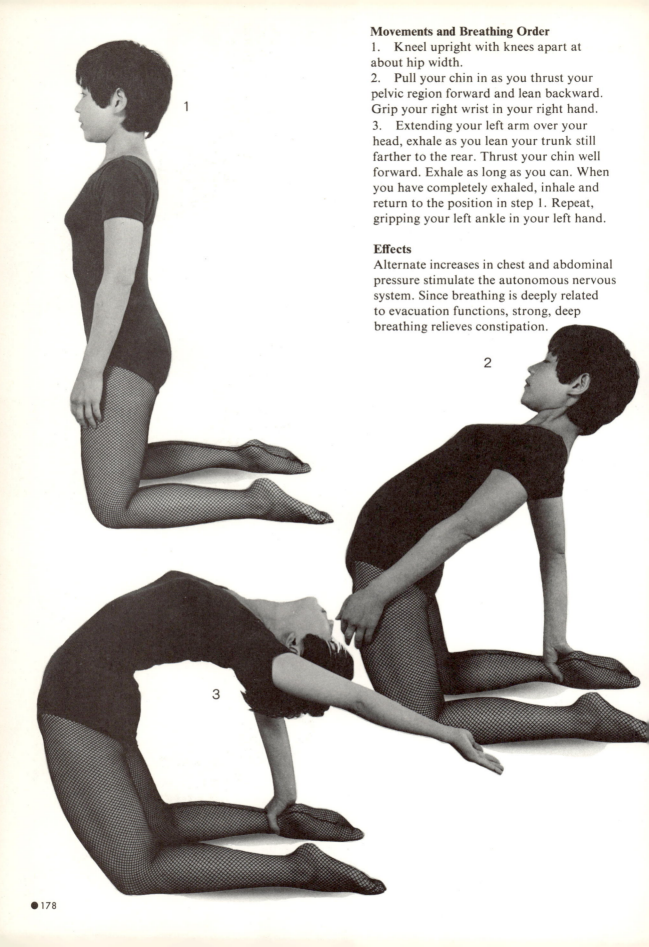

Movements and Breathing Order

1. Kneel upright with knees apart at about hip width.

2. Pull your chin in as you thrust your pelvic region forward and lean backward. Grip your right wrist in your right hand.

3. Extending your left arm over your head, exhale as you lean your trunk still farther to the rear. Thrust your chin well forward. Exhale as long as you can. When you have completely exhaled, inhale and return to the position in step 1. Repeat, gripping your left ankle in your left hand.

Effects

Alternate increases in chest and abdominal pressure stimulate the autonomous nervous system. Since breathing is deeply related to evacuation functions, strong, deep breathing relieves constipation.

Movements and Breathing Order

1. With feet spread wide and body held straight, bend your knees to crouch. Put your hands on your knees.
2. Exhaling powerfully, put your left knee on the floor close to your right heel. At the same time, turn your head rearward to the left.
3. Repeat, putting your right knee on the floor close to your left heel.

Effects

By strengthening the leg muscles, this exercise improves circulation in the abdomen and the functioning of the internal organs. Turning to the left relieves constipation, and turning to the right relieves diarrhea.

1

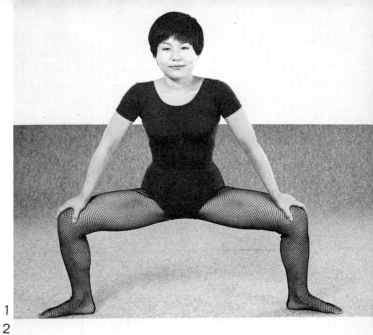

2

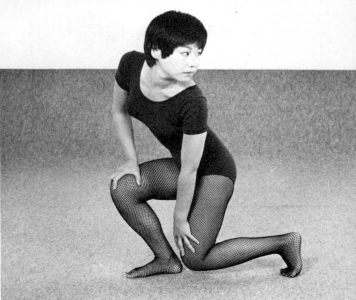

3

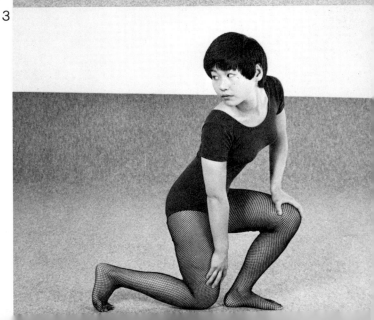

Movements and Breathing Order

1. Lying on your stomach with your legs together, press your forehead firmly against the floor. Then, gripping both ankles from the inside with both hands, exhale slowly as you raise both legs and your trunk. Extend your Achilles' tendons and raise your chin.

2. Exhaling forcefully, pull both feet as if you were attempting to bring them to your head and roll over so that your forehead touches the floor. Inhaling, return to the position in step 1.

Effects

By strengthening the lumbar and abdominal muscles, this exercise relieves constipation and indigestion. In addition, it relieves blood congestion in all the internal organs.

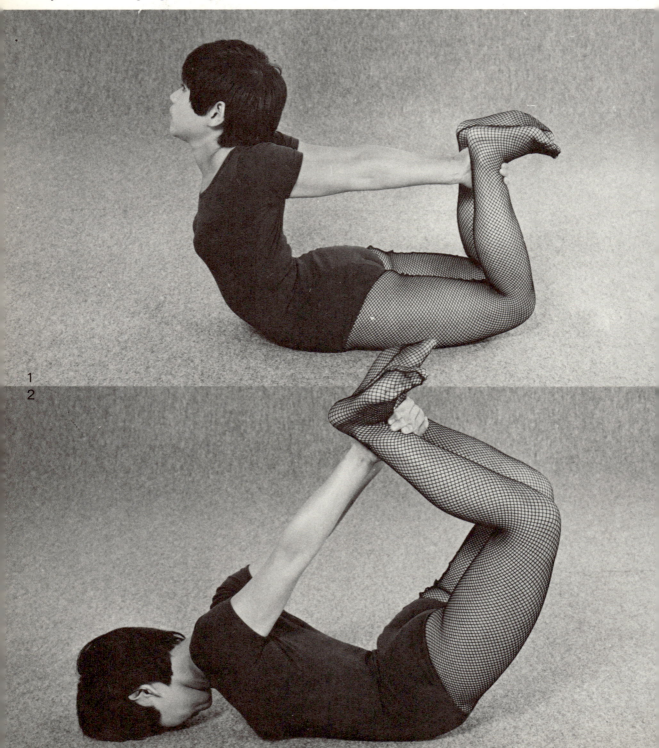

1
2

Movements and Breathing Order

1. Lying on your stomach with both legs together, put your hands on the floor beside your chest. As you inhale deeply, slightly raise your head. Do *kumbhaka* and concentrate strength in your abdomen.

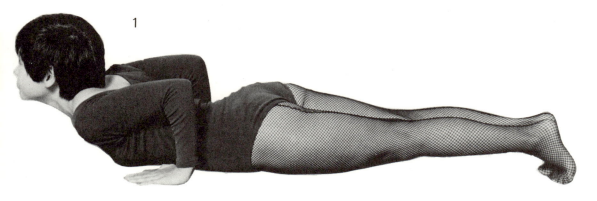

2. Without relaxing your diaphragm, exhale forecefully and raise your upper body. At the same time, bend your knees and lift both legs. Concentrate deliberately on the part of the back that is under greatest pressure. Do *kumbhaka*. As you exhale, raise your trunk still further and bend as far back as possible. When you have exhaled completely, relax, maintaining the same position.

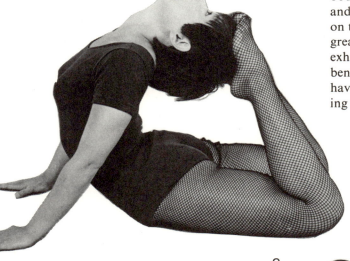

Effects

Since this stimulates the muscles of the back and the abdomen, it has a wholesome, stimulating effect on the internal organs and strengthens the vertebrae.

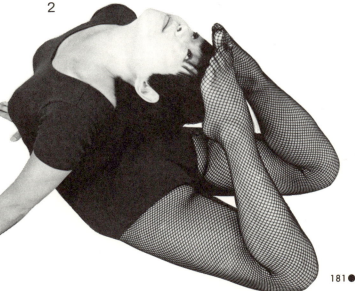

4

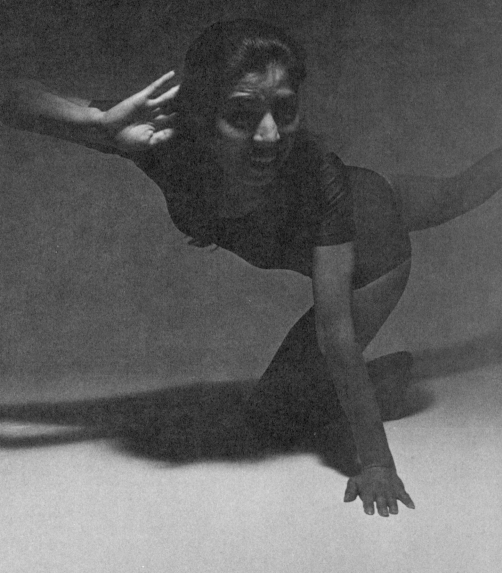

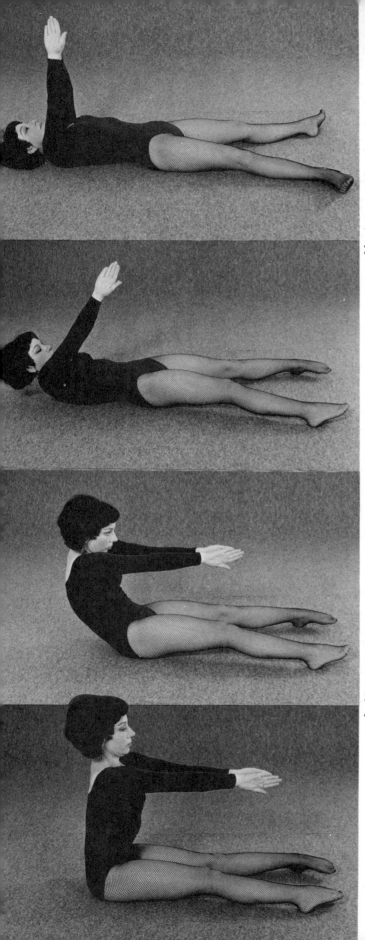

Slenderizing Exercises

Goals and Effects

Overweight people suffer from imbalance in their nervous and endocrine systems. Their malady may be divided into four types: pathological obesity, obesity resulting from incorrect eating, lack of exercise, and incomplete evacuation. In all cases, their rib cages and long bones are expanded and do not close well; and their muscles lack contracting strength. *Yin* foods and too much acid expand and loosen the muscles and internal organs, cause chills, make metabolism sluggish, and stimulate the storage in the body of neutral fats and waste. One of the greatest causes of obesity is excess consumption of sugar and carbohydrates of the kinds found in rice and white bread.

Movement and Breathing Order

1.   Lying on your back with feet spread to about hip width, raise both hands—backs together—straight above your chest.

2.   Turning your big toes inward and bringing them as close to the floor as possible, sit up.

3–4.   Inhale and, as you exhale, turn your feet and hands still further inward. In sitting up, do not try to help yourself by bouncing or by waving your arms.

Effects

By tightening ankles, pelvis, and rib cage, this exercise relieves blood congestion in the internal organs and removes fat from the legs and abdomen.

Movements and Breathing Order ▶

Lying on your back, join both hands behind your neck. Turn your feet inward and bring your big toes together.

2–3.   Join your elbows in front of your face and, turning your feet still further inward and pulling your abdomen in, sit up as you exhale. Inhaling, relax and return to the position in step 1. Repeat.

Effects

Since it tightens the legs and upper chest, this exercise is especially effective in reducing the shoulders and upper chest.

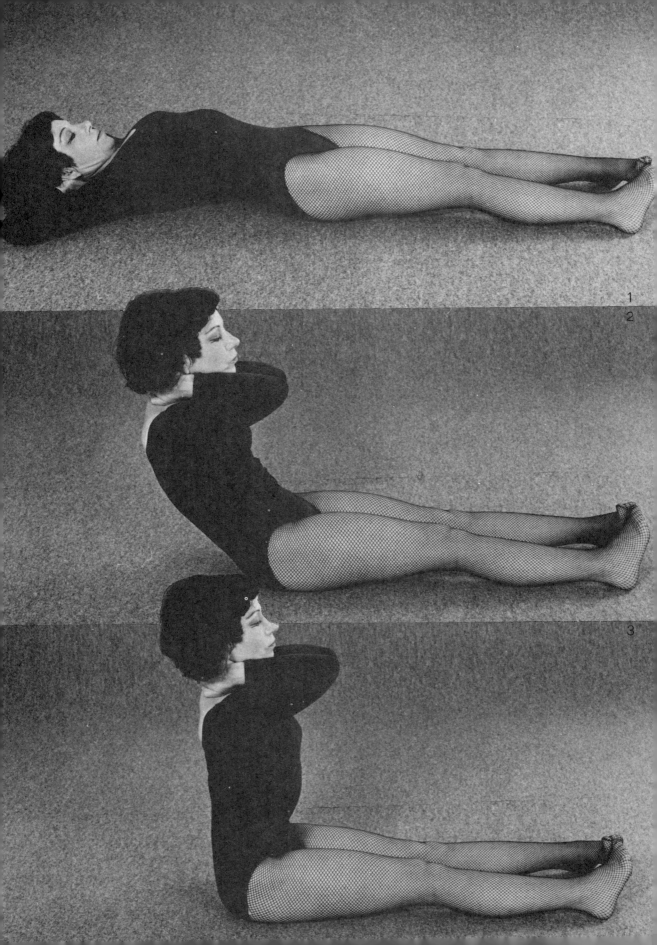

1

2

3

Movements and Breathing Order

1. Lying on your back with both hands behind your neck, turn your feet inward and join your big toes. (This is the same as step 1 in the preceding exercise.)

2. Bring your elbows together in front of your face. Inhale and, as you exhale, raise both your upper body and legs to put your body in a V position. Holding this pose, breathe deeply.

Effects

Because it concentrates strength in the abdomen, this exercise is effective in reducing subcutaneous abdominal fat.

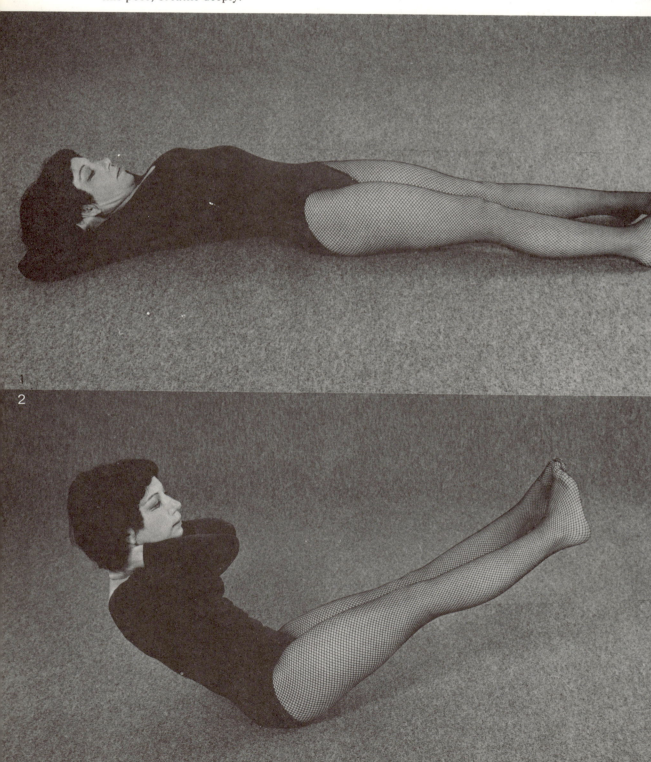

Movements and Breathing Order

1–2. Lying on your back, bend your arms and put your elbows on the floor beside you. Raise your chest. Bring your big toes together and spread your heels.

3. Inhale and, as you exhale, turning your feet further inward, raise and lower your legs. Gradually spread your legs as you repeat this exercise.

Effects

Prolonged overeating causes deposits of fat on the back and resulting round shoulders. This exercise helps cure the overeating habit.

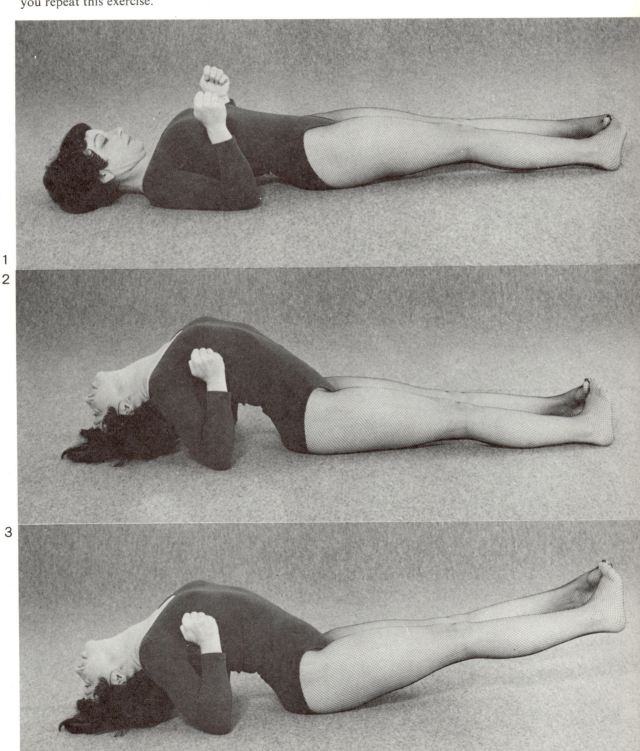

1
2

3

Movements and Breathing Order

1. Sitting cross-legged, bend your elbows, bring your fists to the sides of your chest, and extend your back muscles.
2. Inhale and, as you exhale, put one then the other elbow on the floor behind you.
3. Inhale and, as you exhale, put the top of your head on the floor.
4. As you inhale, raise your knees. Then, as you exhale, lower them close to the floor again. Repeat. Then, exhaling, lower your body.

Effects

Crossing tightens both legs and improves circulation. This exercise removes fat from abdomen and legs.

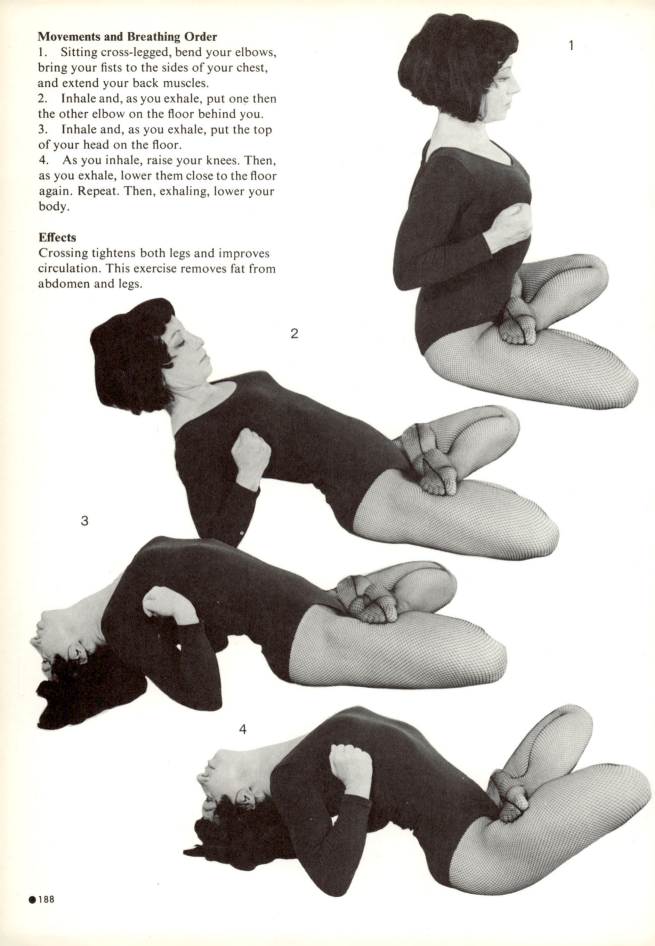

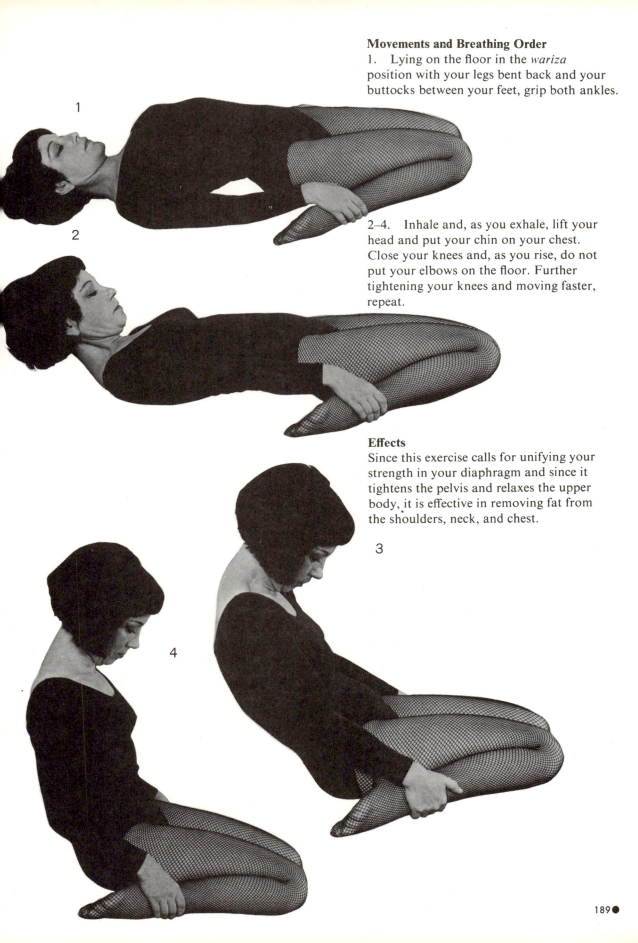

Movements and Breathing Order

1. Lying on the floor in the *wariza* position with your legs bent back and your buttocks between your feet, grip both ankles.

2–4. Inhale and, as you exhale, lift your head and put your chin on your chest. Close your knees and, as you rise, do not put your elbows on the floor. Further tightening your knees and moving faster, repeat.

Effects

Since this exercise calls for unifying your strength in your diaphragm and since it tightens the pelvis and relaxes the upper body, it is effective in removing fat from the shoulders, neck, and chest.

Movements and Breathing Order

1. Sitting with the cross-legged position used in Zen meditation, lean over backward and put the back of your head on the floor. Supporting your body with your arms and elbows, lift your still crossed legs till they are horizontal and your trunk is perpendicular to the floor.

2. Inhale and, as you exhale, raise your legs.

3–4. Inhale and, as you exhale, twist your hips to the right and left.

Effects

Crossing your legs in this way, tightens them and relieves congestion caused in the legs by the standing position. Since this exercise stimulates the thyroid gland, it improves metabolism and removes unwanted subcutaneous fat.

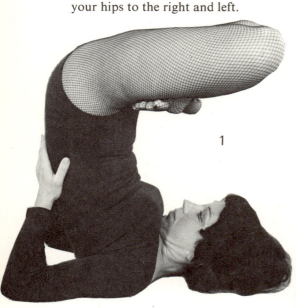

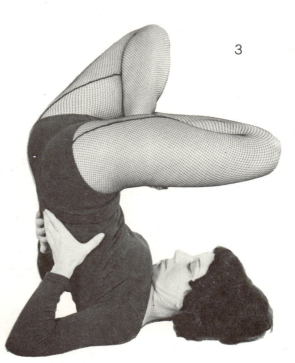

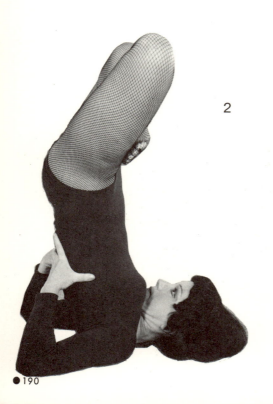

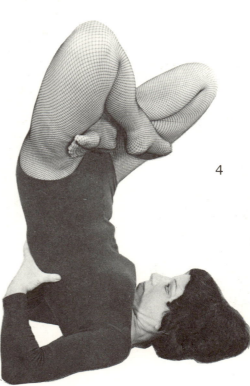

Movements and Breathing Order

1. Lying on your stomach, bend your legs so that only your toes and knees touch the floor and put your hands together, palms down, under your chin (cat pose).

2. Inhale and, as you exhale, swing your hips wide to the right and left. Then, inhaling, return them to the central position (2 A and B). Keep your elbows on the floor and swing your hips as fast as you can.

Effects

Twisting the spine and rib cage stimulates the sympathetic nervous system and tightens the whole body.

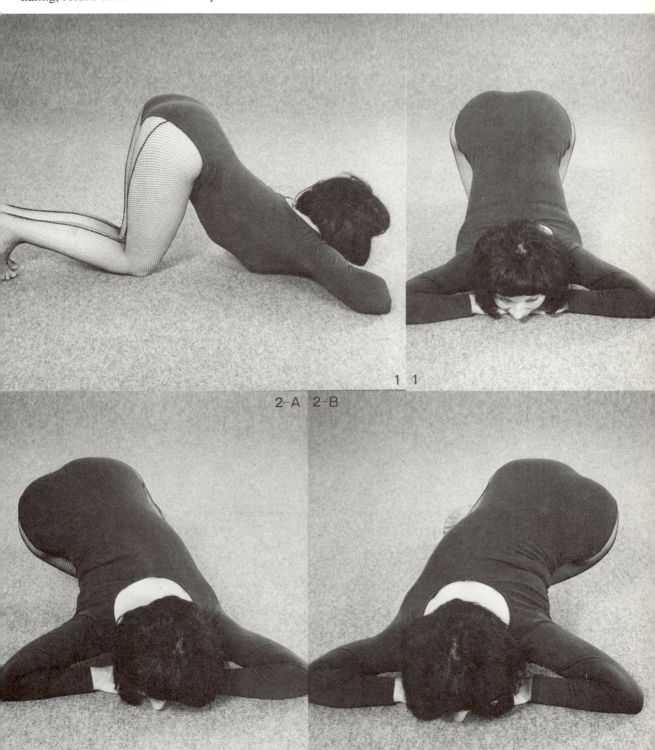

1 1

2-A 2-B

Movements and Breathing Order

1. Lying on your stomach, put your forehead on the floor and grip both ankles from the inside. Keep both knees tight together.

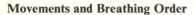

1

2. Inhale and, as you exhale, pull both ankles, raise your legs, and bend your head and upper body to the rear.

3. Inhaling, relax. Then, exhaling, pull harder until you reach maximum force. Keep your knees together.

Effects

This exercise relieves congestion of the blood in the abdomen, tightens the buttocks, and removes fat from the abdomen and buttocks.

2

3

Movements and Breathing Order

1. Lying on your stomach, join both hands, palms outward, behind and above your back.
2. Inhale and, as you exhale, bend your head and upper body back as you lift your hands as high as possible.
3. Holding your upper body in this position, inhale as you turn your toes as far inward as possible. Then, exhaling, raise first one leg then the other.

Effects

Since it tenses them, this exercise removes fat from the buttocks and helps create a higher hip line.

1
2

3
4

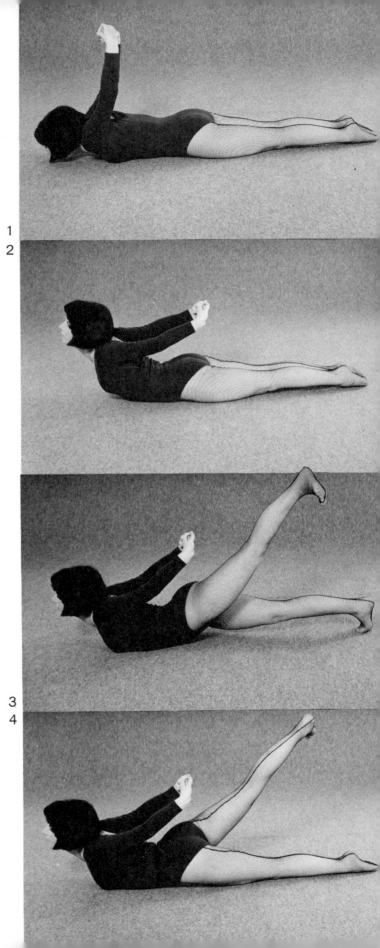

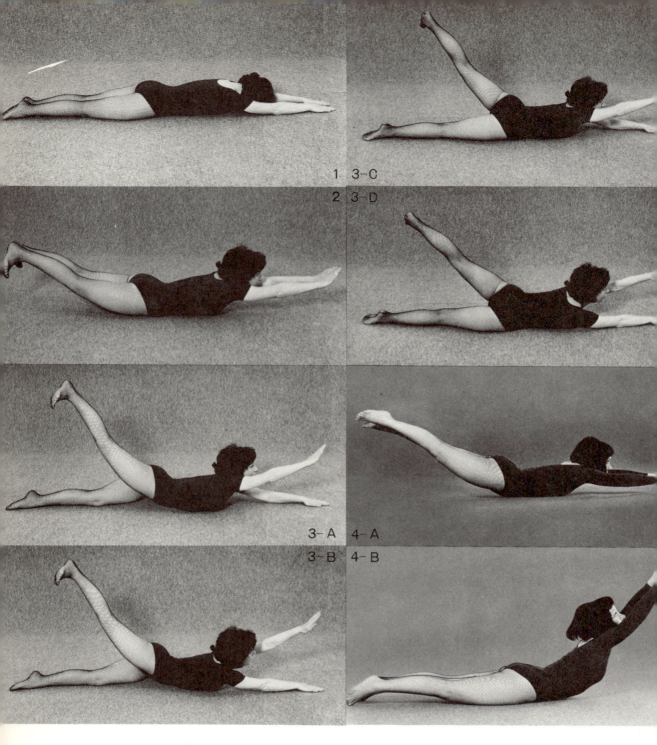

1 3-C
2 3-D
3-A 4-A
3-B 4-B

Movements and Breathing Order

1.   Extend your legs and stretch your arms out on the floor.

2.   Inhale and, as you exhale, raise your arms and bend your upper body and head backward. Raise both legs without bending your knees.

3.   Inhale and, as you exhale, raise your right arm and right leg higher (A) then your left arm and right leg (B). Raise right arm and left leg (C) and left arm and left leg still higher (D). Raise on exhalation and lower on inhalation.

4.   Inhale and, as you exhale, rock forward and backward. (4 A and B). On exhalation, lower your upper body and raise your legs; on inhalation, raise your upper body and lower your legs.

Effects

This relieves congestion in chest and abdomen and tightens buttocks and back.

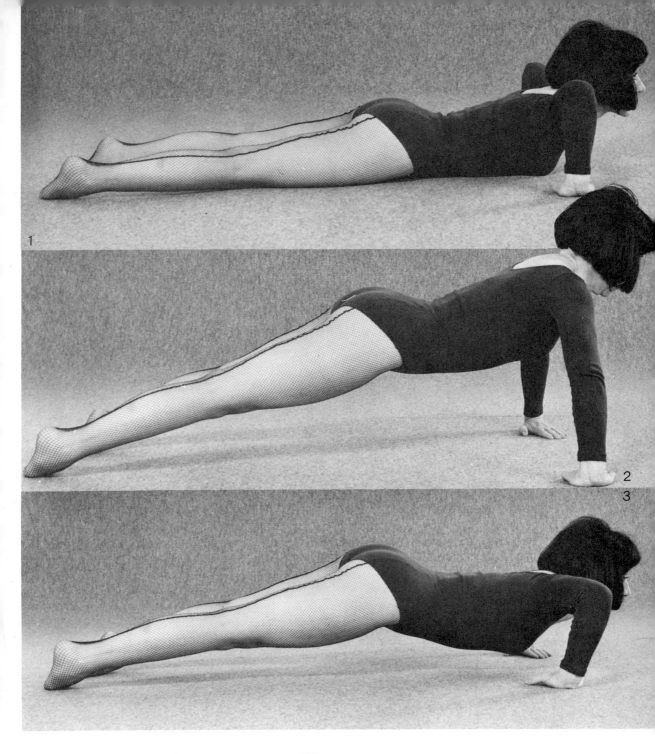

1

2

3

Movements and Breathing Order

1. Lying on your stomach, put your hands—fingers pointed inward—on the floor under your shoulders. With toes turned inward, rest your insteps on the floor.

2–3. Inhale and, as you exhale, rapidly execute push-ups.

Effects

Since the strength of the arms is proportional to the strength with which the rib cage and the pelvis open, this exercise tightens the entire body.

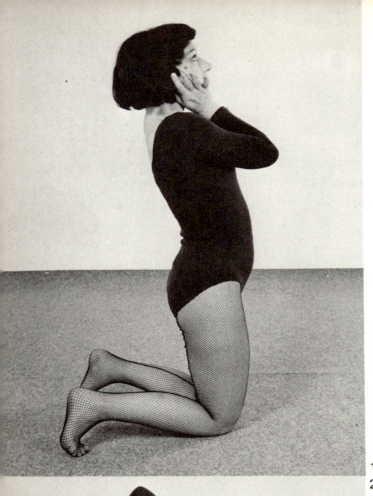

Movements and Breathing Order
1. Kneeling with knees together, toes on the floor, and heels spread, put your hands under your chin and thrust your elbows forward.
2. Inhale and, as you exhale, thrust your hips forward and bend your upper body backward. Inhaling, return to the position in step 1.

Effects
This exercise firms the pelvic region, and the backward bend helps control appetite.

1
2

Movements and Breathing Order ▶
1–2. Standing straight with arms straight to the side, spread your feet about twice as far apart as your hips are wide. Turn the toes of one foot forward and the toes of the other one to the side.
3. Inhale and, as you exhale, taking care that your body does not lean forward, bend straight to the side, raising the opposite hand directly upward. Direct your eyes toward the fingers of the raised hand. Hold this position and breathe deeply.
4. Inhale and, as you exhale, bend still farther to the side until your trunk is parallel with the floor, swing your raised arm to the same side till it too is parallel with the floor. Stretch both arms as far as possible in these directions. Hold this pose and breathe deeply. Then, inhaling, return to the pose in step 1. Repeat, bending in the opposite direction.

Effects
This exercise extends the muscles on the right and left sides and corrects inclination of the pelvis while removing fat from the sides.

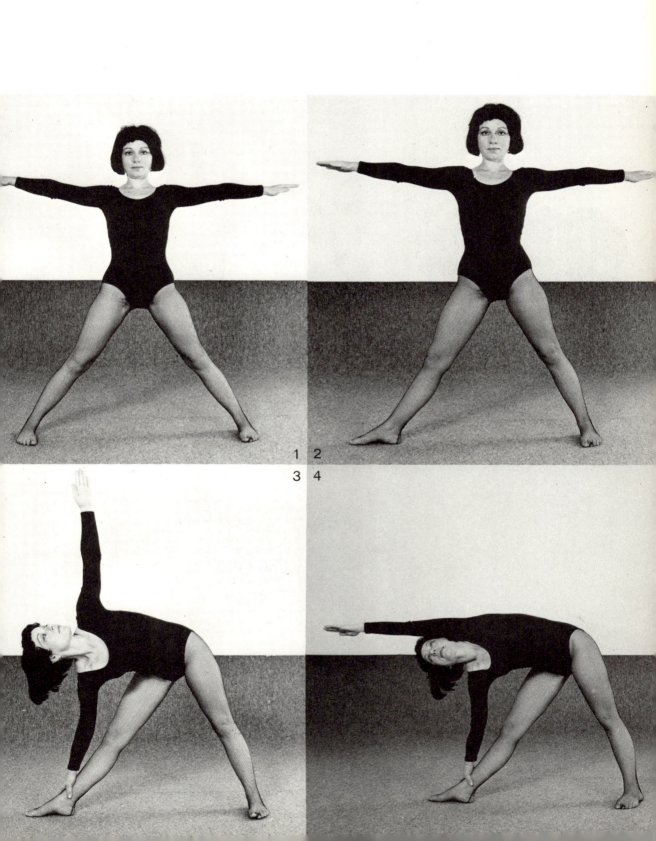

1 2
3 4

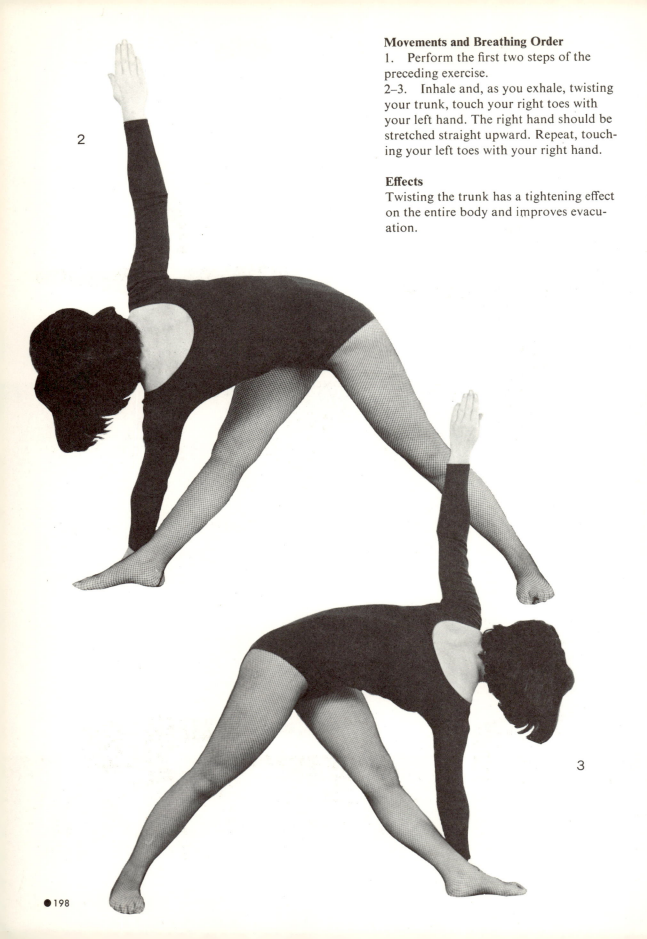

Movements and Breathing Order

1. Perform the first two steps of the preceding exercise.

2–3. Inhale and, as you exhale, twisting your trunk, touch your right toes with your left hand. The right hand should be stretched straight upward. Repeat, touching your left toes with your right hand.

Effects

Twisting the trunk has a tightening effect on the entire body and improves evacuation.

2

3

Movements and Breathing Order

1. Standing with your feet spread about twice as far apart as your hips are wide, put your hands behind your head and extend your elbows to the sides.

2. Inhale and, as you exhale, pivoting on your heels, turn your toes outward and bend your knees. Do not allow your trunk to lean either forward or backward as you lower your hips as far as you can. Once again, pivoting on your heels, turn your toes inward. Inhaling, straighten your knees and return to the position in step 1.

Effects

This exercise tightens the buttocks and develops the chest.

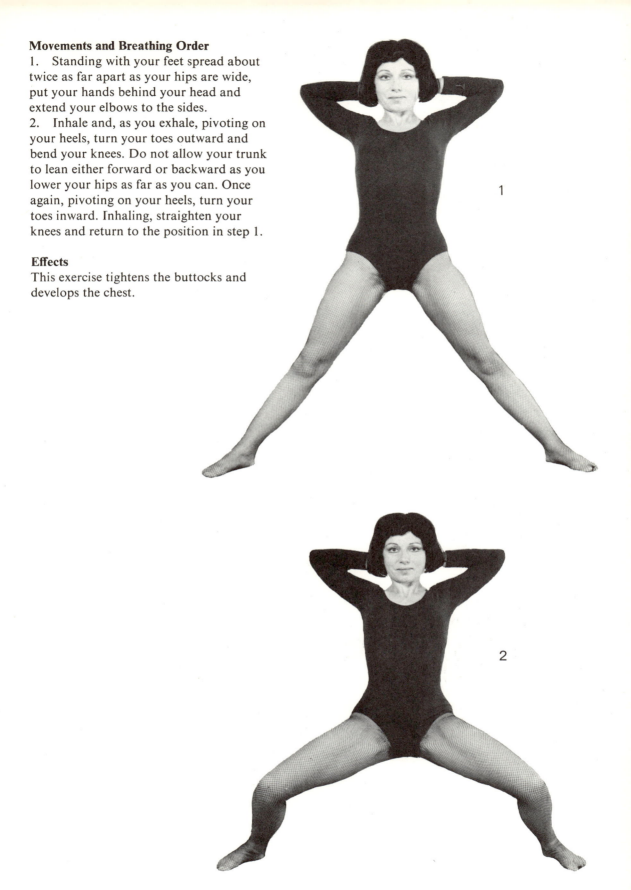

1

2

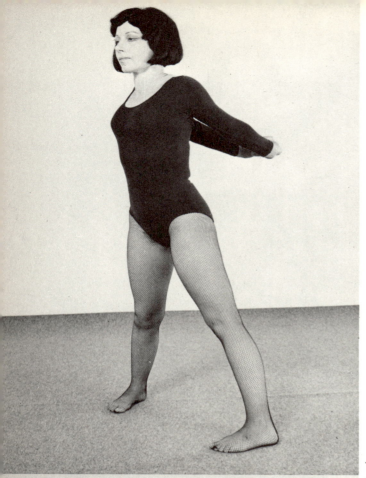

Movements and Breathing Order
Standing straight with feet about as far apart as your hips are wide, join both hands—palms out—well behind your back.

2. Turning your big toes inward, bring your knees together. Inhale and, as you exhale, with knees together, lower your hips as much as possible. Inhaling and still with knees together stand then return to the position in step 1.

Effects
This exercise tightens the inner sides of your thighs and removes fat from the back.

1
2

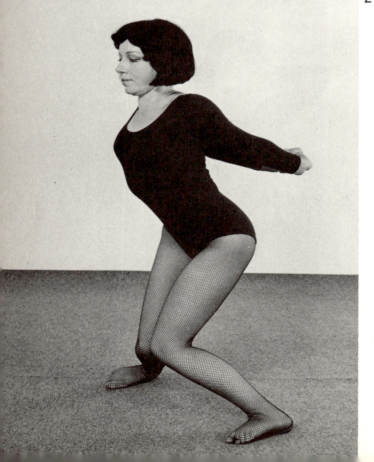

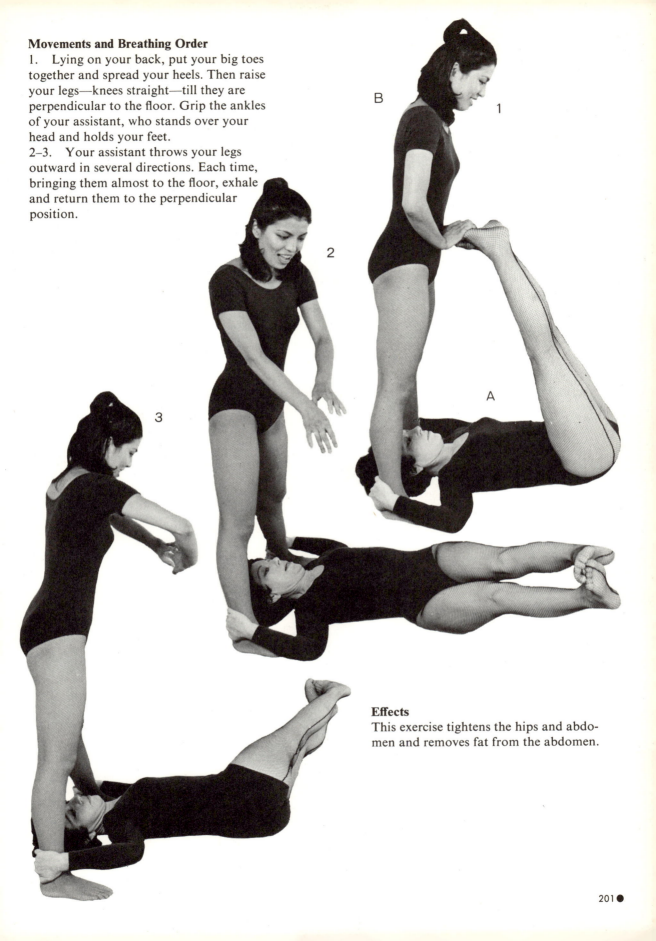

Movements and Breathing Order

1. Lying on your back, put your big toes together and spread your heels. Then raise your legs—knees straight—till they are perpendicular to the floor. Grip the ankles of your assistant, who stands over your head and holds your feet.

2–3. Your assistant throws your legs outward in several directions. Each time, bringing them almost to the floor, exhale and return them to the perpendicular position.

B

1

2

3

A

Effects

This exercise tightens the hips and abdomen and removes fat from the abdomen.

Movements and Breathing Order

1. Lying on your back, raise your knees and spread your feet about as far apart as your hips are wide. Put your hands on your rib cage as if you were pressing your sides. Your assistant kneels on the floor between your feet and presses against the inner sides of your knees with both hands.

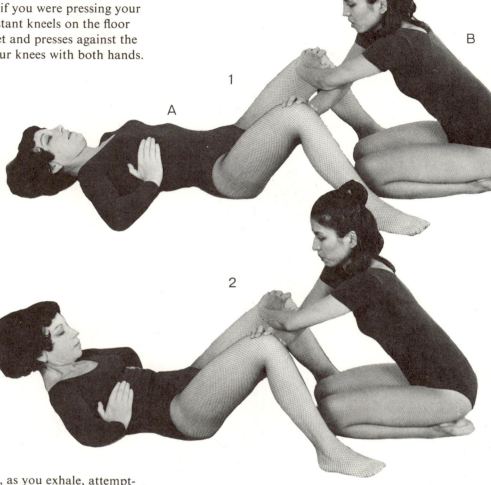

2–3. Inhale and, as you exhale, attempting to close your legs against your assistant's resistance, pull your abdomen in and, pressing your hands against your sides, sit up.

Effects

This exercise improves your ability to close your pelvis.

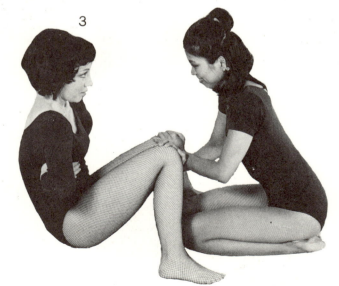

Menstrual Irregularities

Goals and Effects

Immediately prior to and during the menstrual period, women are often tense and highly sensitive in sexually related parts of the body, especially the breasts, which tend to enlarge. Since appetite increases, they often put on weight at these times. In addition, they tend to be sleepy and irritable. As long as the individual experiences no suffering, these are normal symptoms. If irregularities occur only during the menstrual period, they may be overlooked; but if they persist, they should be cured at once, since they can cause other illness. The following exercises are designed to correct twists in the hips, irregularities in the opening and closing of the pelvis, blood congestion in the legs, constipation, and sagging of the buttocks. It is important to train the hips and legs, as well as the abdomen, which tend to be weak in women who suffer from menstrual irregularities. Because psychological elements play a part in these symptoms, meditation increases the effectiveness of the exercises.

Movements and Breathing Order

1.   Lying on your back with your legs outstretched and together, extend your Achilles' tendons. Put your elbows on the floor by your sides, bend your arms, and clench your fists. Raise your chest as high as you can.

2–3.   Inhale and, as you exhale, spread your legs wide and raise and lower them one at a time. Raise them to a height of about thirty centimeters as you inhale and lower them to about five centimeters from the floor as you exhale. Repeat more times on the side on which it is difficult. This exercise is more effective if you open and close your legs as you raise and lower them.

Effects

Raising and spreading your leg stimulates the lateral abdomen.

1

2

3

Movements and Breathing Order

1. Lying on your back with your hands behind your head, put the soles of your feet together and bend your knees.

2. Unbend the knee that is difficult to bend (left in the photograph) and put that foot on the floor. Then, supporting yourself on the toes of that foot and on your head, inhale and, as you exhale, raise that hip.

3. Slowly raise your hip as you exhale and lower it as you inhale. Repeat several times.

Effects

This exercise corrects right-left imbalance in the pelvis and twists in the sacral vertebrae.

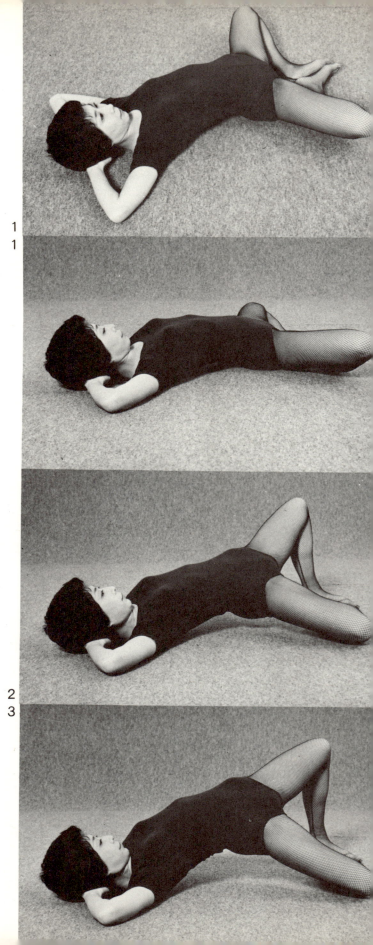

1

1

2

3

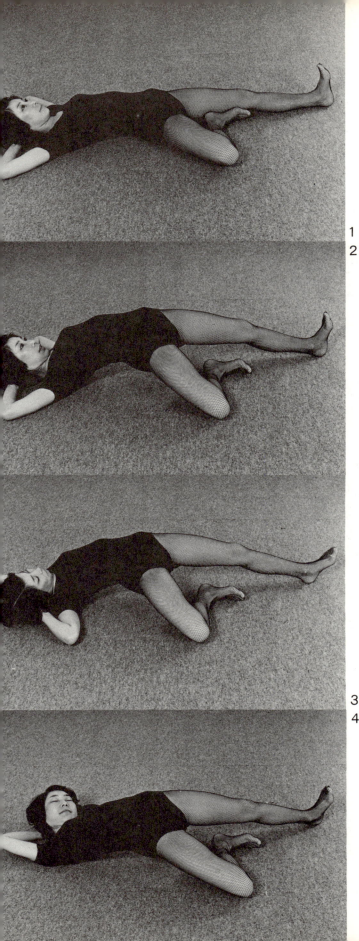

Movements and Breathing Order

1. Lying on your back with both hands joined behind your head and your elbows spread to the side, bend your right knee and bring your right foot to the inner side of your left thigh.

2. Inhale and, as you exhale, put your right knee on the floor and raise your hips as high as you can.

3. Inhale and, as you exhale, twist your trunk to the right and expand your left side.

4. Inhaling, return to the central position. Then bend your trunk to the left. After returning to the central position, slowly lower your hips. Repeat more often on the side on which it is difficult. During the movements in steps 2 and 4, do not let your elbows leave the floor.

Effects

This improves the opening and closing power of the pelvis on the side on which it is contracted and corrects irregular placement of the internal organs.

Movements and Breathing Order

1. Lying on your back, bend your right knee so that your right foot comes to the side of your buttocks and stretch your left leg out straight. Grip your right ankle in your right hand.

2–3. Inhale and, as you exhale, leaving your right knee on the floor and your left leg outstretched, sit up. Inhaling, return to the position in step 1. Repeat, bending the left leg and leaving the right leg outstretched. Execute more times on the side on which it is difficult.

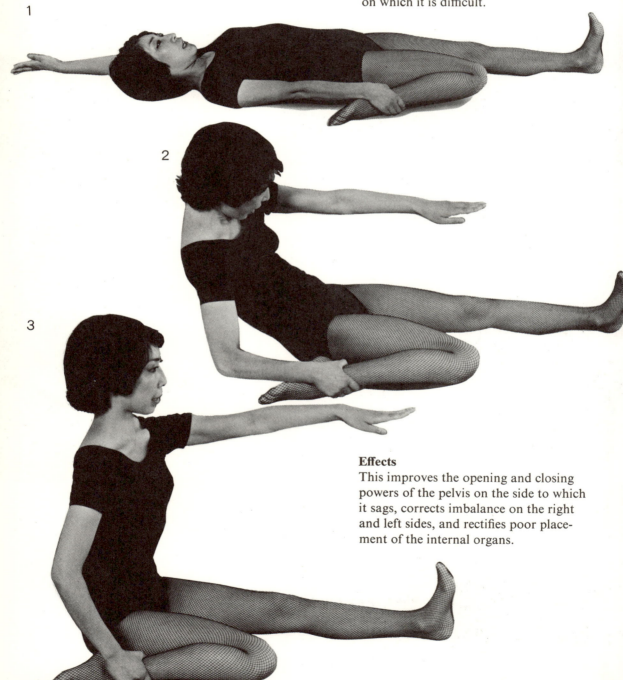

Effects

This improves the opening and closing powers of the pelvis on the side to which it sags, corrects imbalance on the right and left sides, and rectifies poor placement of the internal organs.

Movements and Breathing Order

1. Lying on your back, bend your right knee and grip your right ankle in your right hand. Outstretch your left hand above your head.

2–3. Inhale and, as you exhale, keeping both knees on the floor, swinging your left hand forward, sit up. Repeat, gripping your left ankle in your left hand. It is permissible to have an assistant hold your knees on the floor.

Effects

This exercise corrects twists and differences in the ability of the pelvis to open to one side or the other.

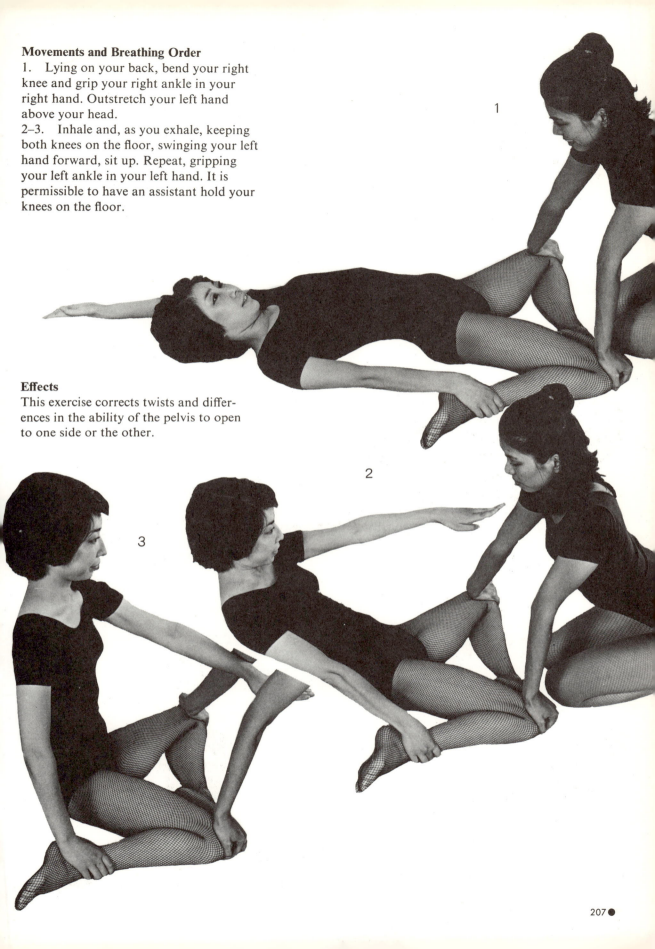

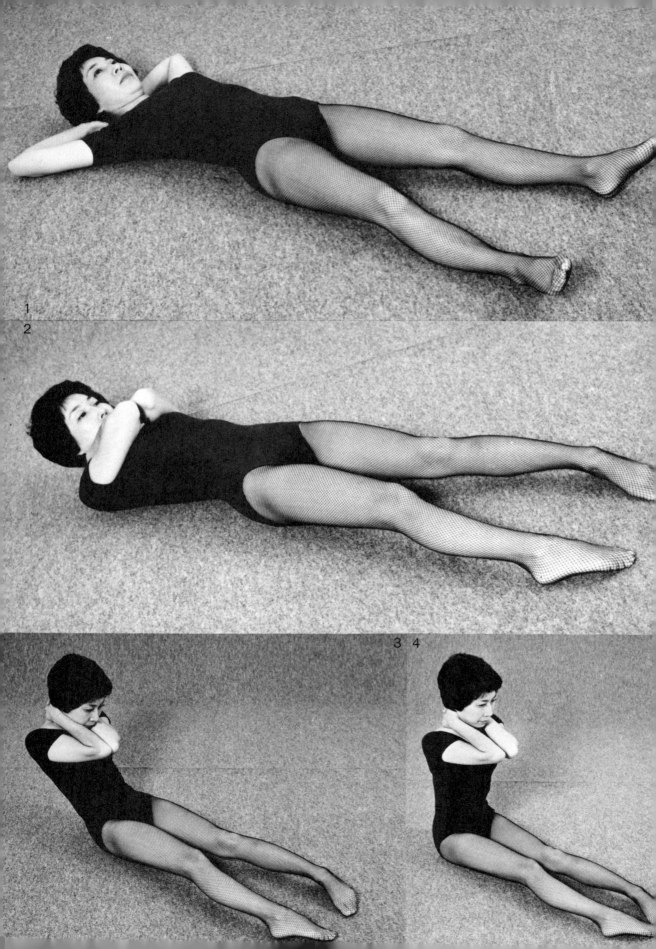

1

2

3 4

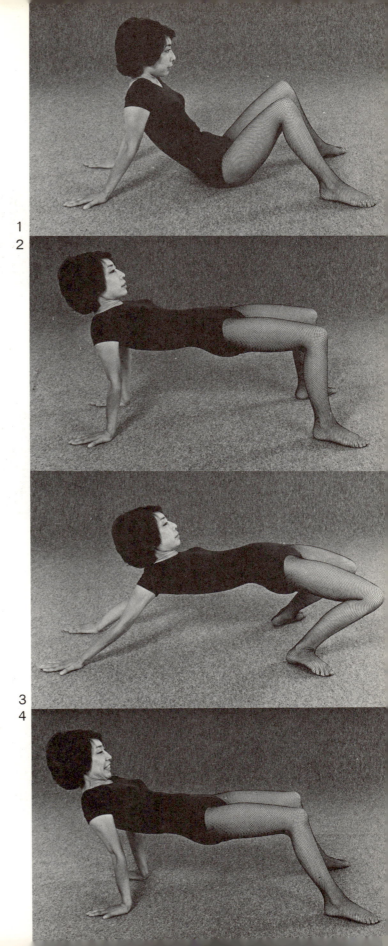

◄ Movements and Breathing Order

1.　Lying on your back with your hands joined behind your head, point your feet inward and put your big toes on the floor.

2–4.　Bring your elbows together and inhale. Then, as you exhale, pull your abdomen in and sit up.

Effects

This tightens the ankles and improves circulation in the legs and lower abdomen. It further removes stiffness of the shoulders and stabilizes the autonomous nervous system.

1
2

Movements and Breathing Order ►

1.　Sit on the floor with your knees raised, your feet about hip width apart, and your hands on the floor behind you.

2.　Inhale and, as you exhale, raise your hips until your body is horizontal and your legs from the knees down and your arms are perpendicular to the floor.

3.　Inhale and, as you exhale, keeping it horizontal, swing your body as far forward as you can.

4.　Inhaling, return to the position in step 2. Then, exhaling, swing your body to the rear. Repeat the movements in 3 and 4 then slowly lower your hips to the floor.

3
4

Effects

This exercise strengthens the hips and abdomen and corrects muscle irregularity and malplacement of the pubic bone.

Movements and Breathing Order

1. Lying on your stomach, put both elbows together on the floor directly below your chin.

Effects

By concentrating strength in the back of the head and the hip region and thus strengthening these parts of the body, this exercise improves blood circulation to the sexual organs and corrects blood congestion in the lower abdomen.

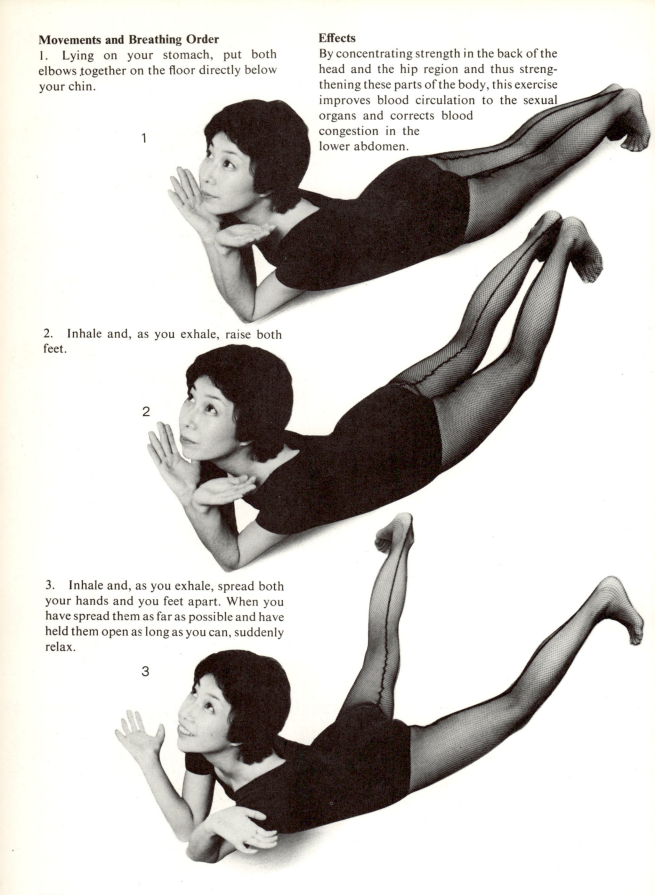

2. Inhale and, as you exhale, raise both feet.

3. Inhale and, as you exhale, spread both your hands and you feet apart. When you have spread them as far as possible and have held them open as long as you can, suddenly relax.

Movements and Breathing Order

1. Crouch with knees and left hand on the floor and with your right hand behind your head and your right elbow extended to the side.

2. Inhale and, as you exhale, twist your hips downward to the left. Inhaling, return them to the central position.

3. Exhaling, slowly twist them downward to the right. Inhaling, return them to the central position. Repeat in the opposite direction with your left hand behind your head and your right hand on the floor.

Effects

This exercise limbers the sides of the abdominal region and corrects twists in the hips.

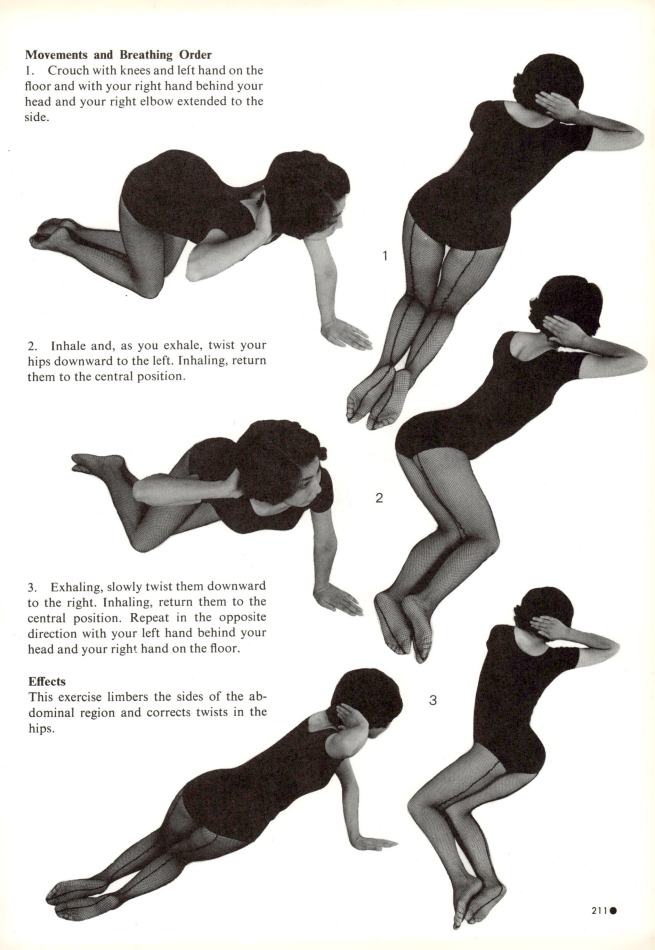

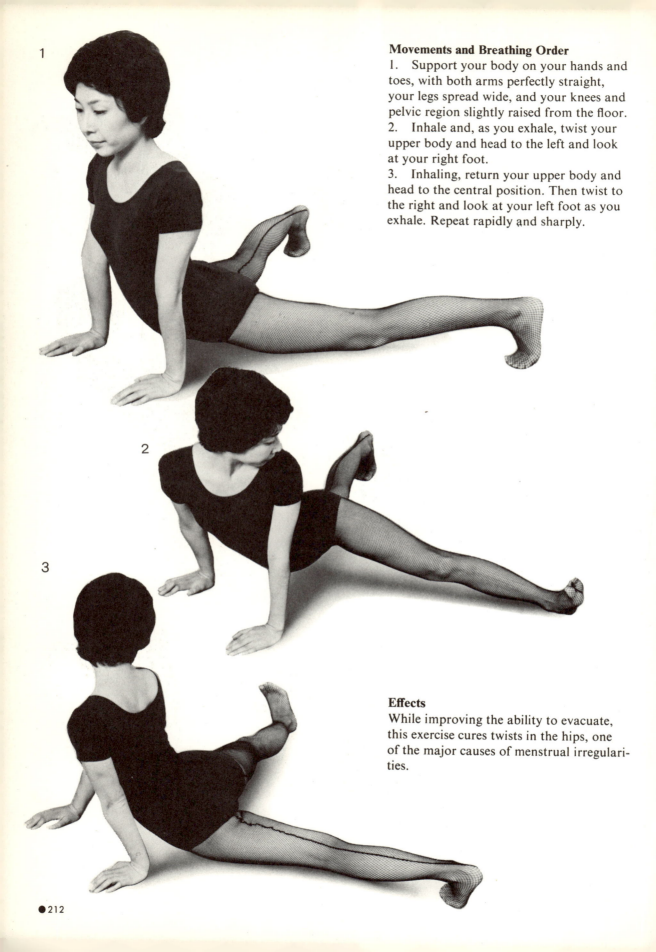

Movements and Breathing Order

1. Support your body on your hands and toes, with both arms perfectly straight, your legs spread wide, and your knees and pelvic region slightly raised from the floor.
2. Inhale and, as you exhale, twist your upper body and head to the left and look at your right foot.
3. Inhaling, return your upper body and head to the central position. Then twist to the right and look at your left foot as you exhale. Repeat rapidly and sharply.

Effects

While improving the ability to evacuate, this exercise cures twists in the hips, one of the major causes of menstrual irregularities.

Easy Childbirth

Goals and Effects

Pathological symptoms experienced in
conjunction with pregnancy are usually
the outcome of such bad habits and ordinary sicknesses as poor diet, constipation, lack of exercise, obesity, overeating,
and excessive use of drugs. Yoga exercises
are designed not only to relieve symptoms
and discomfort associated with these
conditions, but also to influence the entire
life system to prevent the recurrence of
the habits that brought them about. They
encourage natural delivery by correcting
right and left imbalances in the pelvis and
rib cage, improving the tone of the muscles, and stimulating natural breathing.
In addition, they devote special attention
to diet, exercise, natural evacuation, and
powers of neutralization, since these are
intimately related to morning sickness and
other inconveniences of pregnancy. It is
especially important to avoid constipation.
Furthermore, care must be taken to promote a stable emotional and mental state.

Movements and Breathing Order

1.   Sitting on the floor with your hands
joined behind your neck, your chest expanded, and your elbows extended, put
the soles of your feet together and bring
them as close to your body as you can.
2.   Inhale and, as you exhale, bring your
elbows together. At the same time, bring
your knees together.
3.   Inhale and, as you exhale, thrusting
your chest forward, open your elbows as
wide as you can. Repeat. If one of your
elbows is harder to open outward than
the other, pay special attention to opening
it as wide as you can.

Effects

Exercising the elbows and knees improves
the opening and closing abilities of the
pelvis and rib cage.

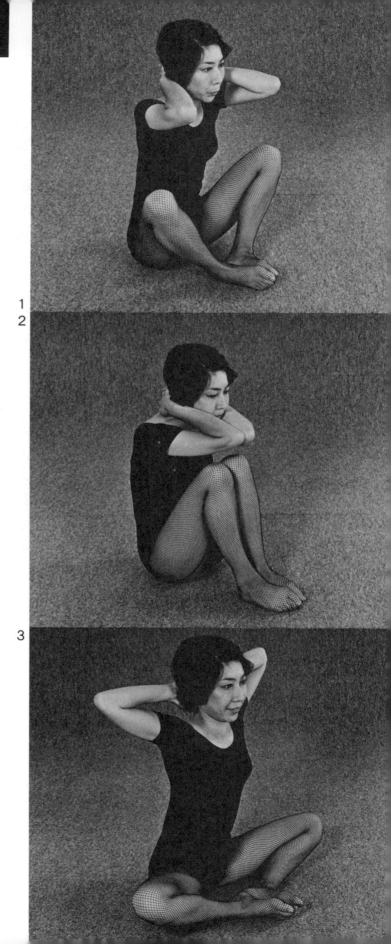

1
2

3

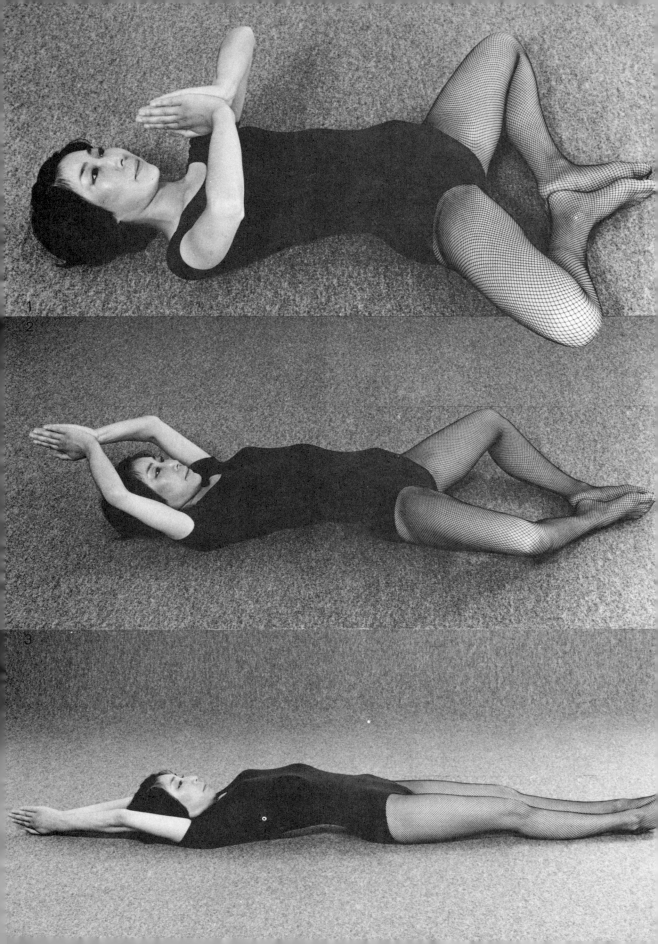

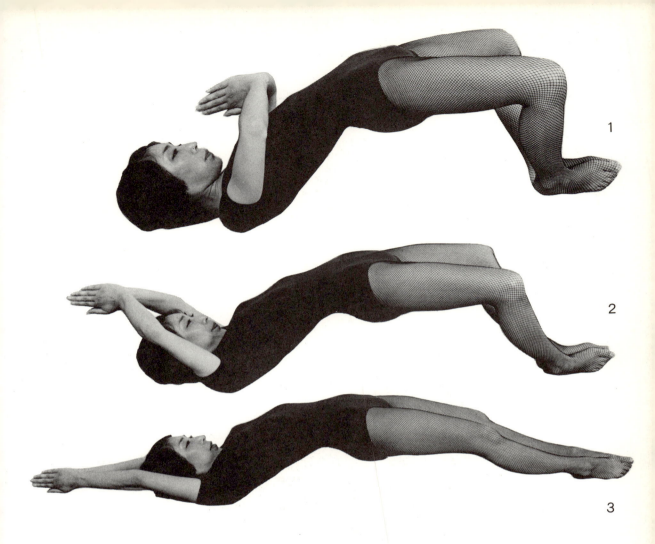

◄ Movements and Breathing Order

1.   Lying on your back with your hands together above your chest, put your soles together and lower your knees to the floor.

2–3.   Inhale and, as you exhale, raise your joined hands above your head. At the same time, with soles joined and feet slightly off the floor, slowly extend your legs. Inhaling, return to the posture in step 1. Repeat several times, gradually increasing speed. If, in step 1, one of your knees is high, put it on the floor and, extending both arms to the side, as you exhale, raise your hips off the floor. Inhaling, bring them close to the floor. Repeat several times (see p. 43).

Effects

The motions performed with hands joined regulate the rib cage; the ones performed with the soles of the feet joined regulate the pelvis. This exercise improves the abdominal muscles and improves breathing.

Movements and Breathing Control

1.   From the position in step 1 of the preceding exercise, inhaling and, as you exhale, open your knees to the sides and raise your hips off the floor.

2–3.   Inhale and, as you exhale, with hips raised, slide your feet forward and extend your arms above your head. Inhaling, return to the position in step 1. Repeat several times then slowly lower your hips to the floor.

Effects

A more strenuous version of the preceding, this exercise strengthens the abdominal muscles.

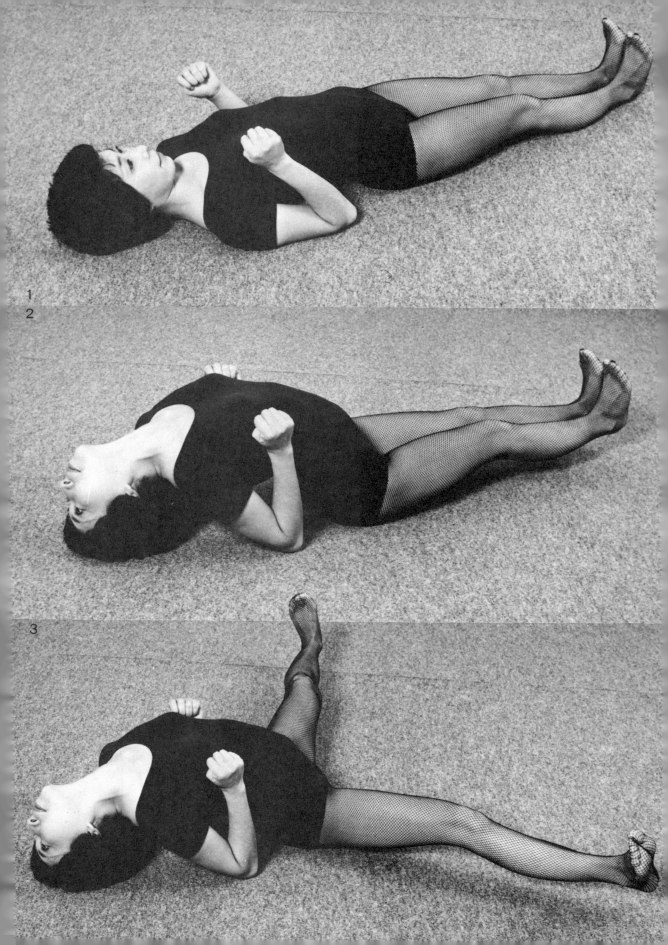

1

2

3

◀ Movements and Breathing Order

1. Lying on your back with your arms bend, elbows on the floor, and fists clenched, extend your Achilles' tendons.
2. Inhale and, as you exhale, raise your chest. Lift your legs slightly off the floor.
3. Spreading your legs, exhale. Inhale as you close them again. Repeat.

Effects

This exercise corrects contraction of the chest and abdominal muscles caused by forward-stooping posture and, by extending and stimulating the lumbar and sacral vertebrae, relieves congestion of blood in the lower abdomen.

Movements and Breathing Order ▶

1. Lying on your back with both hands joined behind your neck and elbows extended to the sides, bend your knees.
2. Bring the heel of your right foot to the base of your left thigh.
3–4. Inhale and, as you exhale, lift your hips from the floor. As you inhale, lift your right knee from the floor. Lower it as you exhale. Repeat several times then slowly lower your hips to the floor. Repeat, putting your left heel at the base of your right thigh.

Effects

Repeating this exercise on the side on which the knee is hard to bend corrects right-left displacement of the pelvis and twists of the hips.

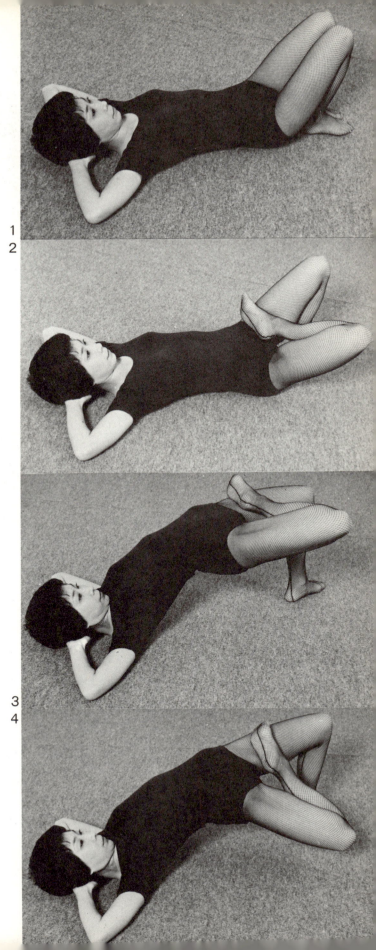

1
2

3
4

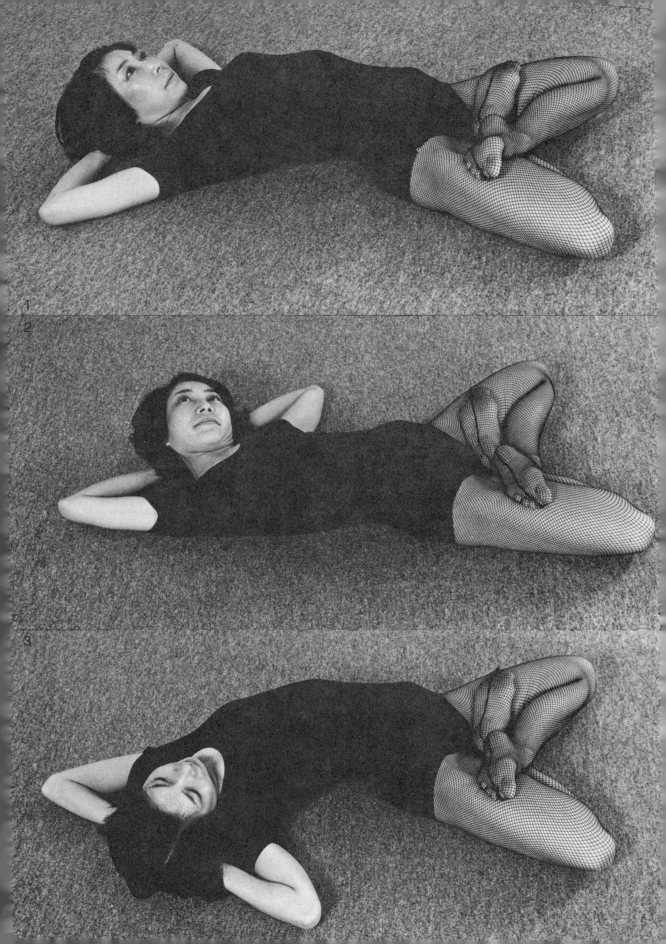

1

2

3

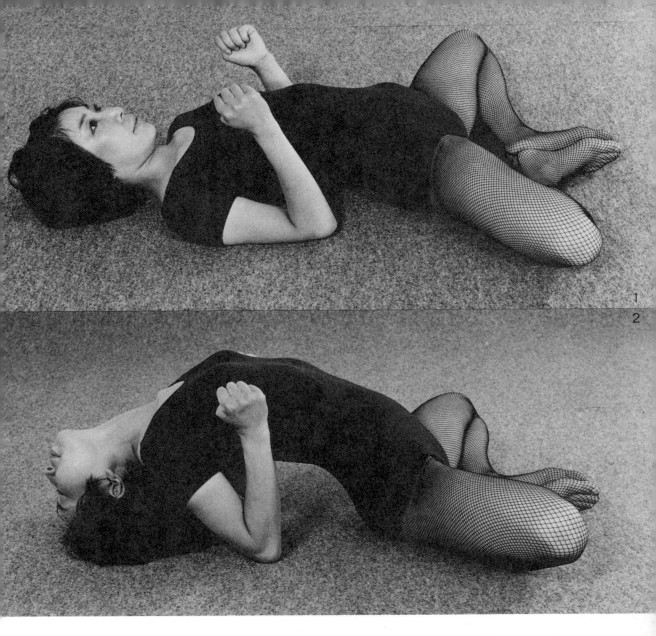

◄ **Movements and Breathing Order**

1. After assuming to meditation pose, lean back till you are lying on the floor with your hands joined behind your head and your elbows extended to the sides.

2. Inhale and, as you exhale, with both elbows still extended to the sides, slide your trunk to the left and thus stretch the muscles of your right side.

3. Inhale, return to the position in step 1, then repeat the exercise in the opposite direction. In bending, bring your elbow and knee as close together as you can.

Effects

Bending your body right and left relieves contractions of the sides and regulates the rib cage.

Movements and Breathing Order

1. Lying on your back, with elbows on the floor, arms bent, and fists clenched, put your soles together and bring them close to your body.

2. As you exhale, open your knees further and, pressing your elbows against the floor, raise your chest. When it is as high as it can go, inhaling, lower it. Then, exhaling, raise it again. Repeat.

Effects

This relieves contraction in the chest, corrects sagging of the rib cage, and tightens the hips. Opening the knees relieves blood congestion in the lower abdomen and contraction of the inner parts thighs.

219●

Movements and Breathing Order

1. Lying on your stomach with both hands on the floor beside your chest, bend both knees outward and bring the soles of your feet together.

2. Inhaling, as you exhale, thrust your chest forward and bend your upper body back. Inhaling, slightly lower your body. Then, exhaling, raise it high again. Repeat.

Then as you inhale, quietly return to the position in step 1.

Effects

This exercise expands and thus relieves contraction and stiffness in the chest and abdominal muscles. In addition, it corrects forward bends in the lumbar vertebrae and increases the flexibility of the spine.

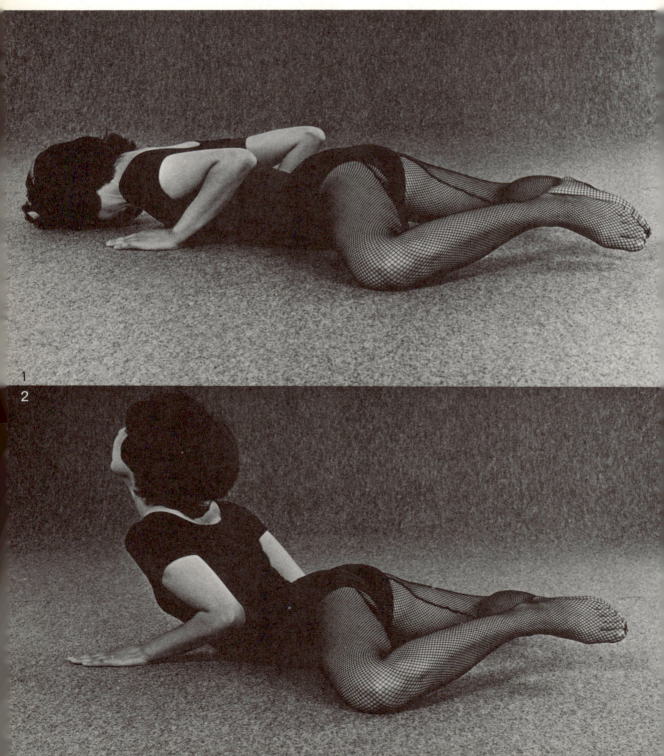

1

2

Movements and Breathing Order

1. Lying on your stomach, bending your arms, and putting your hands on the floor beside your chest, bend your right leg and bring the sole of your right foot to the base of your left thigh.

2. Inhale and, as you exhale, raise your left leg from the floor and bend your upper body upward and back until only the area around your navel remains on the floor. Inhaling, slowly return leg and trunk to the floor. Repeat, bending your left leg. Execute more often on the side on which it is difficult.

Effects

In addition to having the effects of the preceding, this exercise corrects right-left discrepancies in the muscular strength of the hip muscles, adjusts imbalance in the rib cage, and improves the functioning of the kidneys.

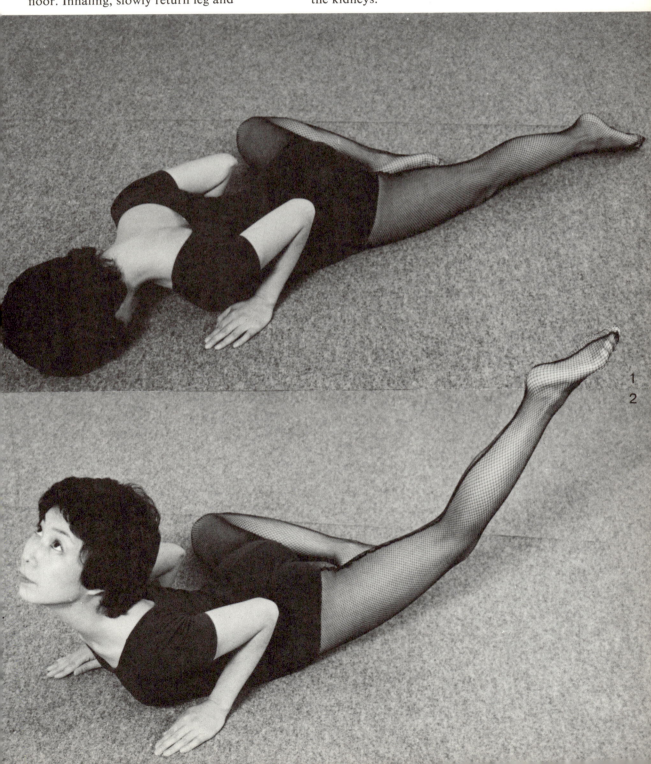

1

2

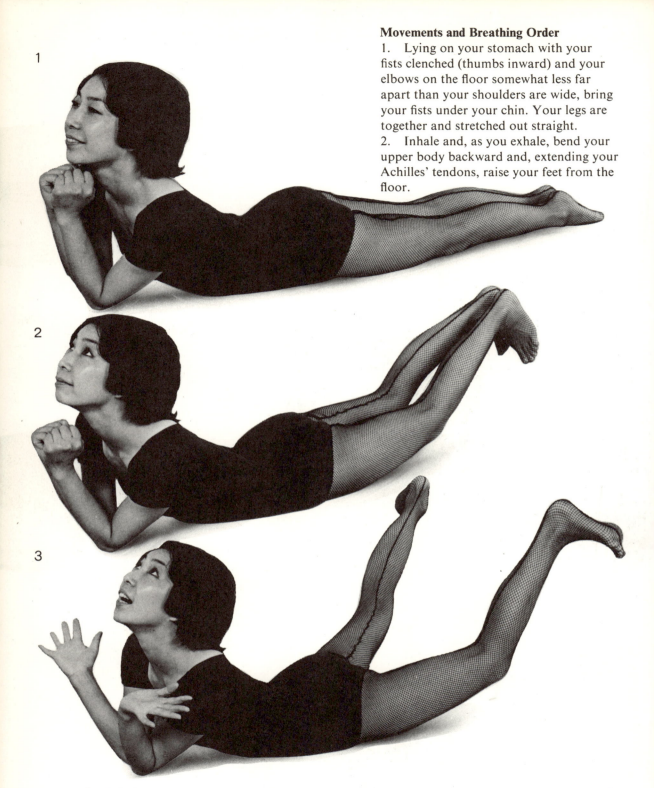

Movements and Breathing Order

1. Lying on your stomach with your fists clenched (thumbs inward) and your elbows on the floor somewhat less far apart than your shoulders are wide, bring your fists under your chin. Your legs are together and stretched out straight.

2. Inhale and, as you exhale, bend your upper body backward and, extending your Achilles' tendons, raise your feet from the floor.

3. Inhale and, as you exhale, spread your legs, which remain raised to the same height as in step 2. Leaving your elbows in the same positions, thrust your chest forward and, spread your hands open and turn both arms outward. Inhaling, slowly and quietly return to the position in step 1.

Effects

Concentrating strength in the rear part of the head and in the hips, this exercise strengthens the hips, relieves blood congestion in the abdomen, corrects inclination of the pelvis, and strengthens the kidneys.

Movements and Breathing Order

1. Lying on your back with both arms extended straight to the sides and both legs spread wide, inhale.

2-3. As you exhale, extending your arms still further to the sides, raise your upper body, chest first. Do not allow your arms to advance farther forward than the shoulder line. If necessary, you may have an assistant hold your feet.

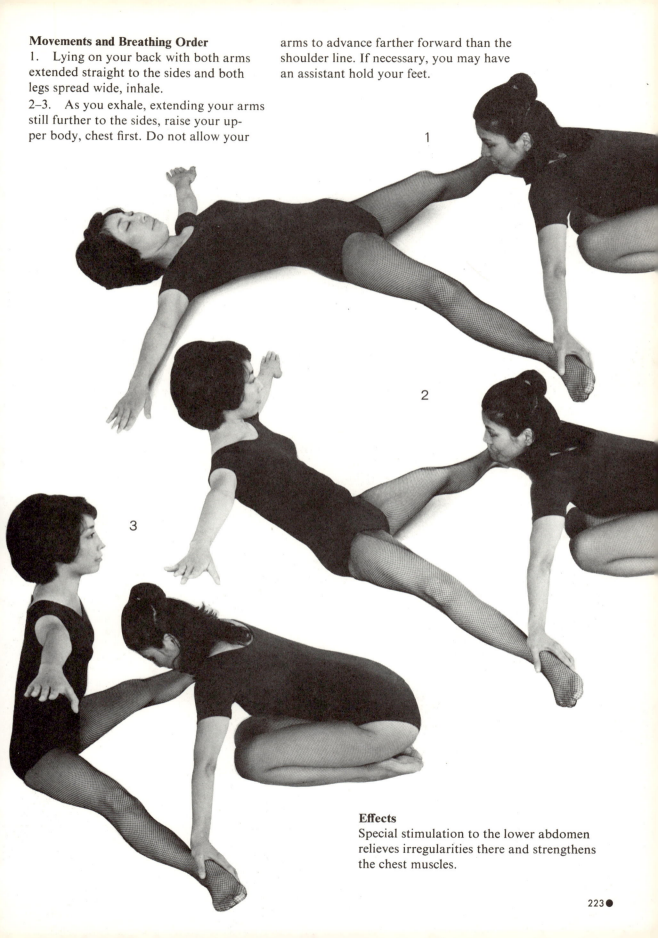

Effects

Special stimulation to the lower abdomen relieves irregularities there and strengthens the chest muscles.

Movements and Breathing Order

1. Lying on your back, bring the soles of your feet together and join the backs of your hands above your abdomen. If necessary, you may have an assistant hold your feet.

2–3. Inhale and, as you exhale, open your knees still farther to the side and sit up. Inhaling, slowly return to the position in step 1.

4–6. Repeat, each time spreading your feet about ten centimeters farther apart.

Effects

This helps develop the muscular strength needed in childbirth.

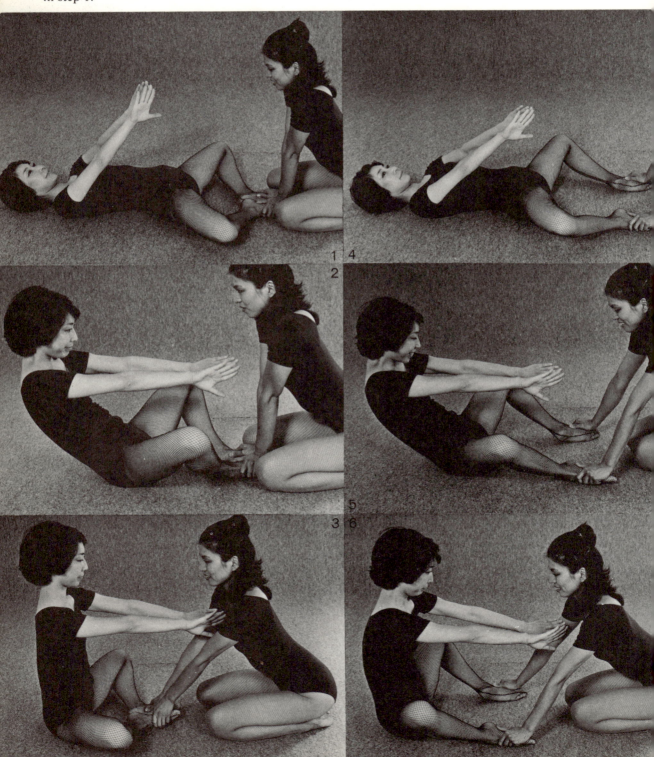